**Misra & Burrill**
**QBASE Radiology 3**

Passing the Fellowship of the Royal College of Radiologists Part 1 examination is a pre-requisite for any doctor who wants a career in radiology. The Part 1 examines candidates' knowledge on both the physics of medical imaging and the principles of radiation protection. This book provides a series of multiple choice questions, structured in a format similar to the examination, in order to evaluate candidates' knowledge on all the aspects that are required for Part 1. The radiation protection questions are up to date with the current IR(ME)R 2000 regulations. Detailed answers, with additional information are provided, along with references, for each question.

The text is accompanied by a free CD-ROM containing the powerful and easy-to-use QBase interactive MCQ examination package. This allows the user to sit the pre-set exams as printed in the book, or to create their own exams using questions drawn from the total pool available on the CD-ROM. The program can either generate these exams randomly, maintaining the same proportions of each subject as the 'pre-set' exams (and the real examinations themselves), or the user can select any number of questions in any subject area to create their very own customised exam to suit their examination practice and the length of time available for each revision session. However the user chooses to set an exam, they can then mark, analyse and store each attempt, review and re-sit the same exam at a later date and compare their scores with previous attempts. When re-sitting an exam, the user can also choose to 'shuffle' the question leaves A–E, making it impossible simply to remember 'patterns' of true and false answers. A final, unique aspect of the program is that it allows the user to select how confident they are of their answer, and the program can then provide feedback on an individual user's 'guessing strategy'.

A brand new feature of this title is that the MCQs are also supplied for use on the Palm (TM) hand-held PDA, allowing the user to practise their MCQs in the ward, in the common room, or even on the bus! This gives a whole new level of flexibility to the acclaimed QBase software.

RAKESH MISRA is Consultant Radiologist at Wycombe Hospital.

JOSHUA BURRILL is Specialist Registrar in Radiology at Central Middlesex Hospital.

# QBASE RADIOLOGY 3
## MCQs FOR THE PART 1 FRCR

**Rakesh Misra, B.Sc. (Hons.), F.R.C.S., F.R.C.R.**
*Consultant Radiologist*
*Wycombe Hospital*
*Buckinghamshire Hospitals NHS Trust*


**Joshua Burrill B.Eng., M.B., B.S., M.R.C.S.**
*Specialist Registrar in Radiology*
*Central Middlesex Hospital*
*North Thames Radiology Rotation*

QBase developed by
Edward Hammond

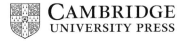

CAMBRIDGE
UNIVERSITY PRESS

CAMBRIDGE UNIVERSITY PRESS
Cambridge, New York, Melbourne, Madrid, Cape Town, Singapore, São Paulo

CAMBRIDGE UNIVERSITY PRESS
The Edinburgh Building, Cambridge CB2 2RU, UK

Published in the United States of America by Cambridge University Press, New York

www.cambridge.org
Information on this title: www.cambridge.org/9780521673839

First published 2006

Printed in the United Kingdom at the University Press, Cambridge

*A catalogue record for this publication is available from the British Library*

ISBN-13: 978-0-521-67383-9 paperback
ISBN-10: 0-521-67383-6 paperback

Every effort has been made in preparing this publication to provide accurate and up-to-date
information which is in accord with accepted standards and practice at the time of publication.
Although case histories are drawn from actual cases, every effort has been made to disguise the
identities of the individuals involved. Nevertheless, the authors, editors and publishers can make
no warranties that the information contained herein is totally free from error, not least because
clinical standards are constantly changing through research and regulation. The authors, editors
and publishers therefore disclaim all liability for direct or consequential damages resulting from
the use of material contained in this publication. Readers are strongly advised to pay careful
attention to information provided by the manufacturer of any drugs or equipment that they
plan to use.

# Contents

# Preface

The first FRCR examination expects candidates to have gained a knowledge of radiation physics, to understand the principles of diagnostic X-ray and radionuclide equipment and the various UK legislation affecting the use of ionising radiations in the medical environment.

No minimum period of clinical experience or clinical radiology training needs to have been completed in order to enter the examination nor is confirmation of course attendance required. (*www.rcr.ac.uk*)

The Part 1 examination comprises a single paper of 25 multiple-choice questions, of 1¼ hours in duration. **QBase Radiology 3** provides 10 sample MCQ papers based on this new exam format, complete with annotated and referenced answers. **QBase Radiology 3** aims to allow a candidate to practice and perfect their examination technique prior to sitting the Part 1 examination. It is aimed at first year radiology registrars and doctors keen to obtain numbers in radiology, where having the Part 1 FRCR is definitely an advantage when it comes to short-listing and interviews.

This new version of QBase includes up-to-date questions on radiation protection, with particular reference to the Ionising Radiations Regulations 1999 and Ionising Radiation (Medical Exposure) Regulations 2000.

RRM was lead author on the previously successful self-assessment books, **QBase Radiology 1** and **QBase Radiology 2**. **QBase Radiology 3** is ideally suited to the new exam format and adds a new innovative Palm-OS™ software-based testing program to allow self-assessment 'on the move'. JB found the previous versions of QBase, with their testing programs, very helpful in the latter stages of his revision. The authors hope that you too will find the experience rewarding.

R.R.M.

J.B.

July, 2005

## INSTALLATION INSTRUCTIONS (CD-ROM VERSION)

### QBase Radiology on CD-ROM

### MINIMUM SYSTEM REQUIREMENTS

- An IBM compatible PC with a 80386 processor and 4MB of RAM
- VGA monitor set up to display at least 256 colours
- CD-ROM drive
- Windows 95 or higher with Microsoft compatible mouse

**NB:** The display setting of your computer must be set to display "SMALL FONTS" (see MS Windows manuals for further instructions on how to do this if necessary)

### INSTALLATION INSTRUCTIONS

The program will install the appropriate files onto your hard drive. It requires the QBase CD-ROM to be in installed in the CD-ROM drive (usually drives D: or E:).

**In order to run QBase, the CD must be in the drive**
Print **Readme.txt** and **Helpfile.txt** on the CD-ROM for fuller instructions and user manual

### WINDOWS 95, 98, 2000, XP

1. Insert the QBase CD-ROM into the drive
2. From the Start Menu, select the Run... option, type **D:\setup.exe** (where D: is the CD-ROM drive) and press OK or **OR** open the contents of the CD-ROM and double-click the **setup.exe** icon
3. Follow the "Full – install all files" to accept the default directory for installation of QBase
4. Click 'Yes' to the prompt "Do you want setup to create Program Manager groups?" If you have a previously installed version of QBase, click 'Yes' to the next prompt "Should the new Program Manager groups replace existing duplicate groups?"
5. To run QBase, go to the Start Menu, then Programs, QBase and **QBase Exam**. From Windows Explorer, double-click the **QBase.exe** file in the QBase folder on your hard drive.

## INSTALLATION INSTRUCTIONS (PALM™ VERSION)

*(See also file Palm installation instructions.doc and .pdf on CD-ROM)*
**MCQ Base** is an application for a Palm™-based PDA. It allows users to test themselves on specific MCQ databases. I wrote it originally prior to my FRCR part 1 to quiz myself on the medical physics and radiation protection parts of the exam.

This is a beta version of the program (v.0.9.0). So far I have not been able to find any bugs in the program and have tested it on both monochrome and colour displays without any problems. However, please remember that it is a program written by a doctor, not a professional programmer and therefore bugs are bound to exist.

The **Qbase Radiology 3 – MCQs for the FRCR Part 1** CD contains the MCQ Base application as well as the FRCR Part 1 MCQ database for it.

### INSTALLATION

The CD contains two files, in the directory PALM, **MCQB**, the MCQ Base application, and **FRCR-Part1**, the MCQ database file. These need to be copied into the system memory of the Palm™. The application will not work if it is copied onto a memory card e.g. SD card.

This assumes the user has a Palm™ PDA with the HotSync cradle and appropriate **Palm Desktop** software, as supplied with the Palm™ PDA, installed on a computer.

To install the necessary components to run MCQ Base for the FRCR Part 1, all one needs to do is double-click on the **MCQB** application and on the **FRCR-Part1** database and this will add these files to a queue ready to be installed on the Palm. Once this has been done a simple **HotSync** of the Palm will transfer the files onto the PDA.

If this however fails, open the **Install Tool** application (part of the **Palm™ Desktop**) and use the *Add ...* button to add **MCQB** and **FRCR-Part1** to the file list. It is important that *All Palm File Types* is selected in the *File of Type* option list, for the application to see both the MCQ Base application and FRCR Part 1 database. Also ensure that the destination is *Handheld* rather than *SD card*. The two parts of the software will then be installed with the next **HotSync** of the Palm.

### USING THE SOFTWARE

MCQ Base is very simple to use. The first screen is a list of available MCQ databases. You should see the following screen.

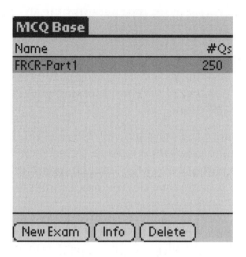

The only MCQ database, **FRCR-Part1**, is already selected. The *Info* button displays a window with information about the selected database. To start a new exam, click on the *New Exam* button, and the following screen appears.

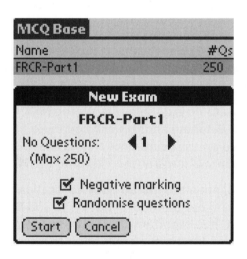

Using the left and right arrows select the number of questions you want to be tested on. If the *Negative marking* check box is ticked then a wrong answer is marked as −1, otherwise a wrong answer is marked as 0. The *Randomise questions* check box allows you to either go through the questions in sequence, or if ticked will provide you with a random set of questions in random order from the entire 250 available.

Once you have selected your choices, pressing the *Start* button starts the MCQ.

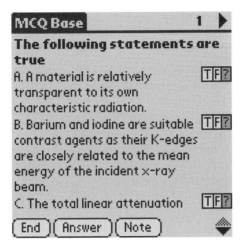

The figure in the top right of the screen is the current question number. The left and right arrows next to this number move you to the next or previous question. The up and down arrows at the bottom right of the screen moves you up and down the different sub-questions from A to E.

To indicate your answer press on the **T**(rue) **F**(alse) **?**(Don't Know) boxes next to the question. To display the correct answers press and hold the *Answer* button and the correct answers appear in the ? boxes. The *Note* button brings up a window with explanatory notes about the current question. The *End* button brings up the score dialogue box as below.

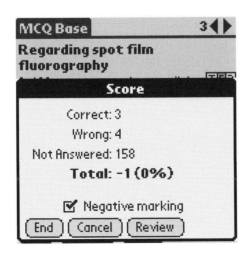

If the *End* button is pressed, then the application returns to the initial screen. However the review button allows you to review your answers as below, and the *Cancel* button returns you to the MCQ quiz without ending it.

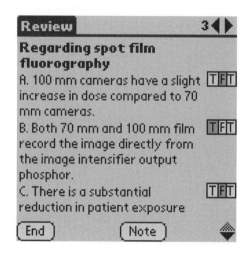

**TROUBLESHOOTING**

Any questions about the software can be emailed to me at palm@burrill.demon.co.uk.

Josh Burrill
*June 2005*

**MCQ Base** © Josh Burrill, 2005

# Notes for users of QBase FRCR on CD-ROM

Please read carefully and print the HELPFILE on the QBase CD-ROM as it contains detailed information on the features and analysis functions of QBase.

QBase is an interactive MCQ examination program designed to help candidates improve their performance in negatively marked MCQs. Please follow the installation instructions printed on the previous page. Once installed, the QBase program resides on your hard disk and reads the data from whatever QBase CD is in your CD drive. If you install QBase from this CD, it will update any previous version of the program. Owners of previous QBase titles will then have access to any new functions available on this new version of the program. All Qbase CDs will work with the new program. To check for successful installation of the new program, check the Quick Start Menu screen: it should have 6 exam buttons.

QBase Radiology 3 contains 250 questions for the new syllabus Part 1 FRCR. The 'Autoset Exam' option on this CD will present you with an exam of 25 questions, utilising any of the 250 questions on the CD. The 10 predefined exams on the CD are constructed in the same way, and are exactly the same as the 10 exams printed in this book. **Please note that there are only 6 exam buttons on the 'Quick Start Menu' screen.** To access exams 7–10 you must go to the 'Main Menu' screen and select the 'Resit exam' option. From the dialogue box that appears, select the 'exam' directory of the **QBase CD in your CD drive** and then choose the exam number you wish to attempt. You can generate your own customised exams using the 'Create your own exam' option. You can save completed exams and your responses to your hard disk, allowing you to review or resit the same paper at a later stage in your revision. Please refer to the helpfile on the CD for more information. To further enhance your revision, instead of selecting the 'Resit exam' option, we suggest that you try the 'Resit shuffled exam' option. The leaves within each question will then be randomly shuffled, removing your ability to remember the pattern of correct answers rather than the facts. The exam analysis functions of QBase will provide you with a detailed breakdown of your performance.

# List of Abbreviations

| | |
|---|---|
| AEC | automatic exposure control |
| Bq | becquerel |
| CaW | calcium tungstate |
| CC | characteristic curve |
| CsI | caesium iodide |
| CT | computed tomography |
| DoH | Department of Health |
| DSA | digital subtraction angiography |
| ED | effective dose |
| EL | exposure latitude |
| EMR | electromagnetic radiation |
| FFD | focus to film distance |
| FOD | focus to object distance |
| FWHM | full width at half maximum |
| GM | Geiger-Muller |
| HIDA | aminodiacetic acid |
| HMPAO | hexamethyl propylene amine oxime |
| HSE | Health & Safety Executive |
| HVL | half-value layer |
| HVT | half-value thickness |
| IC | ionisation chamber |
| IF | intensification factor |
| II | image intensifier |
| IRMER | Ionising Radiation (Medical Exposure) Regulations |
| IRR 88 | Ionising Radiations Regulations 1988 |
| IRR 99 | Ionising Radiation Regulations 1999 |
| Kr-81m | krypton-81m |
| kVp | peak kilovoltage |
| LAC | linear attenuation coefficient |
| LiF | lithium fluoride |
| lP/mm | line pairs per millimetre |
| LSF | line spread function |
| M(ARS)R 78 | Medicines (Administration of Radioactive Substances) Regulations 1978 |
| mA | milliampere |
| MAA | macroaggregates |
| MAC | mass attenuation coefficient |
| MRI | magnetic resonance imaging |
| MTF | modulation transfer function |
| NRPB | National Radiation Protection Board |

| | |
|---|---|
| OFD | object to film distance |
| OPG | orthopantomography |
| PET | positron emission tomography |
| PMT | photomultiplier tubes |
| QA | quality assurance |
| RAT | rotating anode tubes |
| RBE | relative biological effectiveness |
| RPA | radiation protection advisor |
| RPS | radiation protection supervisor |
| SNR | signal to noise ratio |
| SR | spatial resolution |
| Sv | Sieverts |
| Tc | technetium |
| Tc-99m | technetium-99m |
| TLD | thermoluminescent dosimeter |
| U-V | ultraviolet |
| WL | window level |
| Wt | tissue weighting factors |
| WW | window width |
| ZnCdS | zinc cadmium sulphide |

# Section 1 – Questions

# THE ATOM

**Q 1. Regarding the structure of an atom**

- **A.** In an electrically neutral atom, the number of neutrons is the same as the number of orbital electrons
- **B.** The atomic mass number (A) of an element is always equal to or greater than its atomic number (Z)
- **C.** An electron is characterised by having no mass and a unit negative charge
- **D.** The binding energy of a K shell electron is greater than an M shell electron
- **E.** Nuclear exchange forces are effective at distances up to 0.001 mm

# X-RAY TUBES

**Q 2. Regarding a rotating anode tube**

- **A.** Cooling is achieved primarily by conduction of heat along the anode stem
- **B.** A self-rectifying circuit may be used
- **C.** Molybdenum is used in the anode stem due to its high thermal conductivity
- **D.** A tungsten-copper alloy is often used to form the target material at the anode
- **E.** A rotating anode tube has approximately the same efficiency of X-ray production as that of a stationary anode tube

# X-RAY INTERACTIONS

**Q 3. The following statements are true**

- **A.** Bone absorbs more radiation than muscle when low-beam energy is used

**B.** The absorption of radiation is greater for soft tissue in close proximity to bone rather than soft tissue distant from bone

**C.** Filters act by removing high-energy radiation whilst leaving low-energy radiation unchanged

**D.** A filter attenuates radiation predominantly by the photoelectric effect

**E.** An example of a compound filter is of several layers of aluminium separated by a non-attenuating material

## IMAGE QUALITY

**Q 4. Radiographic contrast is decreased by**

**A.** Increasing beam filtration

**B.** Reducing the field size irradiated

**C.** Increasing the kV

**D.** Increasing the focus to object distance (FOD)

**E.** Increasing the object to film distance (OFD)

## FILMS AND SCREENS

**Q 5. At a constant mAs, an increase in the kVp will**

**A.** Produce X-rays of increased wavelength

**B.** Increase the effect of scatter on an X-ray

**C.** Increase the amount of scatter produced within the patient

**D.** Increase film contrast

**E.** Increase film blackening

## GAMMA IMAGING

**Q 6. Regarding the Gamma camera**

**A.** The resolution is increased by increasing the number of photomultiplier tubes

**B.** Collimators are not used

**C.** There is a light-tight housing between the crystal and the photomultiplier tubes

**D.** The scintillation crystal consists of pure sodium iodide

**E.** Following a scintillation, light travels predominantly in the forward direction

# MAMMOGRAPHY

**Q 7. Mammography**

A. The radiological differentiation of normal and abnormal breast tissue is dependent upon photoelectric attenuation in the normal breast
B. Maximum image contrast is obtained at photon energies of the order of 45–60 keV
C. The characteristic radiation of a molybdenum target occurs at 17.9 and 19.5 keV
D. For magnification mammography a focal spot of 0.5 mm diameter is normally used
E. A molybdenum filter attenuates the majority of characteristic radiation produced at a molybdenum target

# FILMS AND SCREENS

**Q 8. Regarding photographic density**

A. Photographic density is a measure of the blackness of a film
B. Photographic density can only be measured objectively
C. The useful density range on a diagnostic X-ray film is from 0.25 to 4
D. The film base usually contributes a density of about 0.07
E. The background fog on an unexposed film usually contributes a density of about 0.05

# CT

**Q 9. Comparing gas-filled ionisation chambers and scintillating crystals used as detectors in CT**

A. Ionisation chambers are more sensitive
B. Scintillation crystals provide a linear response to different radiation intensities
C. Ionisation chambers suffer from the phenomenon known as after-glow
D. Scintillation crystals are more reliable and stable
E. The efficiency of ionisation chambers can be improved by using xenon at high pressure as opposed to air

# X-RAY TUBES

### Q 10. Regarding X-ray tube shielding

**A.** It contains oil to lubricate the bearings of the rotor in a rotating anode tube

**B.** It provides support for permanent beam filters at the tube 'window'

**C.** It forms part of the heat pathway

**D.** The maximum permitted leakage of radiation at 1 m from the focal spot should not exceed 1 Gy/h averaged over an area not exceeding 100 cm$^2$

**E.** Expansion of the lubricating oil secondary to overheating will activate the exposure interlock, thus acting as a safety cut-out

# X-RAY INTERACTIONS

### Q 11. Regarding the interactions which result in X-ray production

**A.** Vary with the atomic number of the target material

**B.** Are always the result of an interaction between an electron and an orbital electron

**C.** Includes characteristic radiation

**D.** Are subject to a maximum energy limit related to the energy of the incident electron

**E.** Bremsstrahlung occurs at only discrete energies

# IMAGE QUALITY

### Q 12. The following are true

**A.** The thicker the structure irradiated, the greater the subject contrast

**B.** The greater the difference in linear attenuation coefficients (LAC) between 2 tissues, the less the subject contrast

**C.** Increasing kV increases subject contrast

**D.** Increasing filtration increases skin dose

**E.** Reducing the field size irradiated decreases contrast

# FILMS AND SCREENS

**Q 13. The following statements regarding exposure latitude are true**

   A. Exposure latitude (EL) is the range of exposure factors which will give a correctly exposed image of a subject
   B. EL is independent of subject contrast
   C. EL is dependent on film gamma
   D. EL can be increased by using a lower kV
   E. EL can be increased by using a film of lower gamma

# THE ATOM

**Q 14. Regarding atoms and their structure**

   A. The mass number defines the number of nucleons within an atom
   B. The L shell contains a maximum of 18 electrons
   C. Isotopes of an element have different physical properties
   D. An alpha particle is four times heavier than an electron
   E. An isobar is any nucleus which has the same atomic mass number as another nucleus

# FILMS AND SCREENS

**Q 15. Regarding the metallic replacement method of silver recovery**

   A. This can be used in conjunction with an automated processor
   B. Requires electric power
   C. Uses steel wool
   D. It is possible to reuse the fixer after silver recovery with this method
   E. The silver produced is 90–95% pure metallic silver

# X-RAYS INTERACTIONS

**Q 16. Regarding the photoelectric effect**

   A. The interacting photon disappears completely
   B. This involves the interaction between a photon and a free electron

**C.** Characteristic radiation is produced

**D.** Results in the production of an ionised atom

**E.** As the photoelectron slows down and loses energy, no further ionisation is produced

## DOSIMETRY

Q 17. **Patient dose may be reduced by**

**A.** The use of a bucky grid

**B.** The use of tube filtration

**C.** The use of a high kV

**D.** The use of a lower mA

**E.** The use of a larger focus to film distance

## X-RAY TUBES

Q 18. **Heat loss from an X-ray tube**

**A.** Heat is transferred by conduction from the anode disc to the oil in the tube housing

**B.** Heat is transferred by radiation from the anode disc to the oil in the tube housing

**C.** The oil in the tube housing acts as both an insulator and as a cooling agent

**D.** Heat is transferred by convection through the oil to the tube housing

**E.** Minimal heat is conducted along the anode stem in a rotating anode tube

## GAMMA IMAGING

Q 19. **Regarding positron emission tomography (PET)**

**A.** A positron has a unit positive charge and mass identical to that of an electron

**B.** Positrons tend to be emitted from nuclides with an excess of neutrons

**C.** The scintillation detector is usually made of bismuth germinate

**D.** The emitters that are used in PET imaging generally have long half-lives

**E.** Annihilation radiation occurs resulting in the coincident production of high-energy photons

# RADIATION PROTECTION

## Q 20. The following actions are measures for reducing patient dose

A. Using a fast film screen combination

B. Using low attenuation (e.g. carbon fibre) materials for table tops

C. Using digital radiography equipment

D. Use of gonad shields

E. Use of compression techniques where possible

# RADIATION PROTECTION

## Q 21. Regarding the '10 day rule'

A. Applies to radiography of the skull

B. Should be applied to women who have been taking the oral contraceptive pill for not less than 3 months and found it effective

C. Should be applied to women who have an IUCD for not less than one month and have found it effective

D. Should be applied to women who have been sterilised

E. Should be applied to women who are menstruating at the time of the examination

# RADIATION PROTECTION

## Q 22. Regarding non-stochastic effects

A. All non-stochastic effects are dose dependent

B. Above a threshold dose level, the severity of non-stochastic effects is proportional to the radiation dose

C. Lung fibrosis is an example of a non-stochastic effect

D. Skin necrosis is an example of a non-stochastic effect

E. Diarrhoea is an example of a non-stochastic effect

# RADIATION PROTECTION

## Q 23. The following statements are true

A. The annual whole body dose limit for a patient undergoing treatment is 500 millisieverts (mSv)

B. The equivalent dose limit to the abdomen of a female of reproductive capacity is 13 mSv/year

**C.** Once pregnancy has been declared, the equivalent dose limit to the pregnant abdomen must not exceed 2 mSv for the remainder of the pregnancy

**D.** The whole body annual effective dose limit for staff (18 years and over) is 30 mSv

**E.** The dose limit to the pregnant abdomen is 5 mSv over the term of the pregnancy

## RADIATION PROTECTION

**Q 24. Regarding the exposure to natural background radiation**

**A.** Contributes about 2.2 mSv of the total per caput annual dose

**B.** Is greatest at sea level

**C.** 50% of the total natural background exposure is from radon and thoron emissions

**D.** Contributes ten times the dose as that from occupational exposure

**E.** Food and drink contribute about 300 μSv to the total per caput annual dose

## RADIATION PROTECTION

**Q 25. The following statements are true**

**A.** A controlled area is required where constant exposure to a shielded source would result in 3/10ths of a dose limit being exceeded

**B.** A 'controlled area' is required if the exposure dose rate were to exceed 5 μSv/h

**C.** Areas where the exposure dose rate lies between 2.5 and 5 μSv/h are known as 'supervised areas'

**D.** The radiation protection supervisor is often an experienced physicist

**E.** The radiation protection advisor is often a senior radiographer

# Section 2 – Answers

**A 1.**   **A.** false   **B.** true   **C.** false   **D.** true   **E.** false

In an electrically neutral atom, it is the number of protons that is equal to the number of orbital electrons.

While an electron has a unit negative charge, it has a mass of $9.11 \times 10^{-13}$ kg.

Nuclear exchange forces are effective at only very short distances in the order of $10^{-15}$ m.

Curry, Thomas. *Christensen's Physics of Diagnostic Radiology,* 4th Edn. Williams & Wilkins (Europe) Ltd.

**A 2.**   **A.** false   **B.** false   **C.** false   **D.** false   **E.** true

The principle mode of cooling is via radiation of heat. There is minimal conduction through the anode stem to the bearings.

A full wave rectified circuit is required.

Molybdenum has low heat conductivity; this prevents the passage of heat to the bearings.

A tungsten rhenium alloy is used. This improves the thermal capacity of the anode and resists roughening.

The efficiency of X-ray production in both the rotating and stationary anode tube is about 1%.

Curry, Thomas. *Christensen's Physics of Diagnostic Radiology,* 4th Edn. Williams & Wilkins (Europe) Ltd.

**A 3.**   **A.** true   **B.** true   **C.** false   **D.** true   **E.** false

Filtration removes useless low-energy radiation which contributes to patient dose without contributing to the useful image.

A compound filter usually consists of two or more layers of different materials.

Curry, Thomas. *Christensen's Physics of Diagnostic Radiology,* 4th Edn. Williams & Wilkins (Europe) Ltd.

**A 4. A.** true  **B.** false  **C.** true  **D.** false  **E.** false

Filtration results in beam hardening, and thus reduces contrast.
Reducing the field size reduces the amount of scatter produced,
and thus improves contrast.
Radiographic contrast is independent of the FOD.
Increasing the OFD amounts to using an 'air gap' technique, and in
this setting contrast is increased due to scatter 'missing' the film.

Curry, Thomas. *Christensen's Physics of Diagnostic Radiology,* 4th Edn.
Williams & Wilkins (Europe) Ltd.

**A 5. A.** false  **B.** true  **C.** false  **D.** false  **E.** true

At higher kVp the X-ray emitted is of greater energy which has a
shorter wavelength.
At increased kVp the amount of scatter produced is reduced.
At increased kVp film contrast tends to decrease.

Curry, Thomas. *Christensen's Physics of Diagnostic Radiology,* 4th Edn.
Williams & Wilkins (Europe) Ltd.

**A 6. A.** true  **B.** false  **C.** true  **D.** false  **E.** false

As gamma radiation is emitted in all directions from the patient,
the use of the collimator is intended to match the pattern of
scintillation within the crystal, with the distribution of gamma
emissions from within the patient.
The scintillation crystal consists of sodium iodide with added
thallium impurities.
There is no preponderance for light to travel in the forward
direction. Following a scintillation, light can travel in any direction,
and some light is received by each of the photomultiplier tubes.

Curry, Thomas. *Christensen's Physics of Diagnostic Radiology,* 4th Edn.
Williams & Wilkins (Europe) Ltd.

**A 7. A.** true  **B.** false  **C.** true  **D.** false  **E.** false

The maximum tube voltage for mammography is about 30 kVp
In magnification mammography a very small focal spot diameter
is required; 0.1 mm focal spots are used.
A filter is transparent to its own characteristic radiation.

Armstrong. *Lecture Notes on the Physics of Radiology*, 1st Edn. Clinical Press
Ltd., 1990.

Exam 1

Answers

**A** 8. **A.** true **B.** false **C.** false **D.** true **E.** true

Photographic density can be subjective, as judged by the eye or objective, as measured by a densitometry.
The useful density range is from 0.25 to 2. Densities less than 0.25 are too light to be seen by the human eye, and those greater than 2 are too dark.

Armstrong. *Lecture Notes on the Physics of Radiology*, 1st Edn. Clinical Press Ltd., 1990.

**A** 9. **A.** false **B.** false **C.** false **D.** false **E.** true

Ionisation chambers are less sensitive, produce a linear response to different radiation intensities, do not suffer from after-glow and are more reliable/stable as compared to scintillation crystals.

Armstrong. Lecture Notes on the Physics of Radiology, 1st Edn. Clinical Press Ltd., 1990.

**A** 10. **A.** false **B.** true **C.** true **D.** false **E.** false

The oil within the tube shielding acts as an insulator for the high voltage transformer. The rotor is lubricated with soft metal such as silver.
The maximum permitted leakage is 1 mGy/h at 1 m from the focal spot over an area not exceeding 100 cm$^2$.
Overheating of the oil will activate the tube thermal interlock, thus terminating the exposure. The exposure interlock is activated if:

(i)   there is an incorrect filament supply for the kV selected;
(ii)  there is an incorrect current to the stator for anode rotation;
(iii) there is insufficient time for (i) and (ii) to occur.

Curry, Thomas. *Christensen's Physics of Diagnostic Radiology,* 4th Edn. Williams & Wilkins (Europe) Ltd.

**A** 11. **A.** true **B.** false **C.** true **D.** true **E.** false

Interactions which produce X-rays may be the result of kinetic energy lost by an electron as it is deflected by the positive charge of a nucleus. The energy lost is emitted as photons of radiation. A continuous spectrum of energies is produced. Interactions of electrons with a bound orbital electron produce characteristic radiation.

Bremsstrahlung is a continuous spectrum of energies.

Curry, Thomas. *Christensen's Physics of Diagnostic Radiology,* 4th Edn. Williams & Wilkins (Europe) Ltd.

A 12. **A.** true **B.** false **C.** false **D.** false **E.** false

Subject contrast, C, depends on (a) the thickness, T, of the structure and (b) the differences in LACs of the tissues involved. Hence C is proportional to (LAC 1 − LAC 2) × T.

Increasing kV decreases subject contrast.

Increasing filtration decreases skin dose.

Decreasing the field size reduces the amount of scatter radiation and thus improves contrast.

Farr, Allisy-Roberts. *Physics for Medical Imaging*, 1st Edn. W. B. Saunders Co. Ltd.

A 13. **A.** true **B.** false **C.** true **D.** false **E.** true

With an increase in kV, with mAs reduced to compensate, subject contrast is reduced. This results in some gain of exposure latitude.

Farr, Allisy-Roberts. *Physics for Medical Imaging,* 1st Edn. W. B. Saunders Co. Ltd.

A 14. **A.** true **B.** false **C.** true **D.** false **E.** true

The L shell contains 8 electrons whilst the M shell contains 18 electrons.

An alpha particle is more than 7,000 times heavier than an electron.

Curry, Thomas. *Christensen's Physics of Diagnostic Radiology*, 4th Edn. Williams & Wilkins (Europe) Ltd.

A 15. **A.** true **B.** false **C.** true **D.** false **E.** false

This method involves the use of steel wool only and does not require any electric power.

The fixer cannot be recycled and has to be disposed of.

The silver produced by this method is in the form of a silver sludge which requires refining. However, in the electrolytic method, 90–95% pure metallic silver is obtained.

Curry, Thomas. *Christensen's Physics of Diagnostic Radiology*, 4th Edn. Williams & Wilkins (Europe) Ltd.

**A** 16. **A.** true   **B.** false   **C.** true   **D.** true   **E.** false

In the photoelectric effect the interaction is between a photon and a bound electron.
The photoelectron loses energy by interacting with matter resulting in further ionisations.

Curry, Thomas. *Christensen's Physics of Diagnostic Radiology,* 4th Edn. Williams & Wilkins (Europe) Ltd.

**A** 17. **A.** false   **B.** true   **C.** true   **D.** false   **E.** false

The use of a secondary radiation grid requires an increase in exposure factors, and thus increased dose to the patient.
Filters remove the useless unwanted low-energy photons which do not contribute to the useful image.
The use of a lower mA will result in the need of a compensatory increase in exposure time. Thus the total exposure will remain unchanged.
The number of photons required to produce an X-ray image is independent of the focus to film distance. Hence, the dose is also independent of focus to film distance.

Curry, Thomas. *Christensen's Physics of Diagnostic Radiology,* 4th Edn. Williams & Wilkins (Europe) Ltd.

**A** 18. **A.** false   **B.** true   **C.** true   **D.** false   **E.** true

Heat is transferred by conduction through the oil to the tube housing, and then by convection to the surrounding air.

Curry, Thomas. *Christensen's Physics of Diagnostic Radiology*, 4th Edn. Williams & Wilkins (Europe) Ltd.

**A** 19. **A.** true   **B.** false   **C.** true   **D.** false   **E.** true

Positrons tend to be emitted from nuclides with an excess of protons. A proton is converted into a neutron and a positron.

The radionuclides used in PET imaging have very short half-lives e.g. Fluorine-18 (110 min), Carbon-11 (20.5 min), Nitrogen-13 (10 min), Oxygen-15 (2 min)

Curry, Thomas. *Christensen's Physics of Diagnostic Radiology*, 4th Edn. Williams & Wilkins (Europe) Ltd.

**A** **20.** **A.** true **B.** true **C.** true **D.** true **E.** true

Farr, Allisy-Roberts. *Physics for Medical Imaging*, 1st Edn. W. B. Saunders Co. Ltd.

**A** **21.** **A.** false **B.** false **C.** true **D.** false **E.** false

The '10 day rule' aims at confining less urgent radiological examinations of the lower abdomen and pelvis on females of childbearing age, to the ten days following the start of menstruation. The rule applies to plain radiography and special examinations such as barium enema and HSGs.
The '10 day rule' is not applicable to women who have had an IUCD for not less than 3 months and have found it effective.

*British Journal of Radiology* 1976; 49: 201–202.

**A** **22.** **A.** true **B.** true **C.** true **D.** true **E.** true

Curry, Thomas. *Christensen's Physics of Diagnostic Radiology*, 4th Edn. Williams & Wilkins (Europe) Ltd.

**A** **23.** **A.** false **B.** false **C.** true **D.** false **E.** false

There are no dose limits for patients undergoing treatment. However, ALARA must be practised.
The dose limit to the abdomen of a female of reproductive capacity is 13 mSv per quarter.
The annual effective dose is 20 mSv for staff (18 years of age and over).
The proposed dose limit to the pregnant abdomen is about 2 mSv (<1 mSv to the foetus) over the term of the pregnancy.

*The Ionising Radiation Regulations 1999*

**A 24. A.** true **B.** false **C.** true **D.** false **E.** true

Natural background radiation contributes 85% of the total background exposure. Of this 50% is due to radon and thoron, 12% to food and drink, 13% to gamma rays and 10% to cosmic rays. Artificial exposure contributes 15% of which diagnostic medial radiation is the largest artificial source (14%). Occupational exposure contributes 0.3%. The total per caput annual dose is about 2.6 mSv.

Farr, Allisy-Roberts. *Physics for Medical Imaging*, 1st Edn. W. B. Saunders Co. Ltd.

**A 25. A.** true **B.** false **C.** false **D.** false **E.** false

Controlled area: exposure dose rate >7.5 μSv/h.
Supervised area: exposure dose rate = 2.5–7.5 μSv/h.
The radiation protection supervisor is a senior radiographer.
The radiation protection advisor is an experienced physicist.

Farr, Allisy-Roberts. Physics for Medical Imaging, 1st Edn. W. B. Saunders Co. Ltd.

## FILMS AND SCREENS

**Q 1.** **Intensifying screens**

**A.** Calcium tungstate fluoresces blue light

**B.** The efficiency of production of light with a calcium tungstate screen is 50%

**C.** Lanthanum oxybromide emits green light

**D.** Intensification factor is the ratio of exposure needed with the screen to the exposure needed without the screen

**E.** A film cassette containing a double-sided emulsion film and two intensifying screens, results in doubling of the speed of exposure and also doubling of the resultant film contrast obtained

## FLUOROSCOPY

**Q 2.** **Regarding spot film fluorography**

**A.** 100 mm cameras have a slight increase in dose compared to 70 mm cameras

**B.** Both 70 and 100 mm film record the image directly from the image intensifier output phosphor

**C.** There is a substantial reduction in patient exposure dose compared to film screen techniques

**D.** There is a loss of resolution with spot film compared to film screen techniques

**E.** The exposure time for spot film fluorography is about one quarter to one sixth of that required for a full-size X-ray

## X-RAY INTERACTIONS

**Q 3.** **Regarding coherent scattering**

**A.** It is responsible for the majority of scatter which reaches a film

**B.** Includes Thompson scattering

**C.** Results in a change in the wavelength of the scattered photon

**D.** Does not result in ionisation within the patient

**E.** Accounts for 25% of the interactions in the diagnostic energy range

## X-RAY TUBES

**Q 4.** **Regarding an X-ray tube**

**A.** Bremsstrahlung radiation makes up the majority of the useful beam throughout the diagnostic energy range

**B.** 10% of the total X-ray production occurs as a result of an interaction between filament electrons and M shell electrons in the target

**C.** At 20 keV the photoelectric effect accounts for >50% of the total interactions

**D.** The kVp is responsible for the tube current

**E.** The interaction between an electron from the cathode filament and the target anode produces Bremsstrahlung radiation

## FILMS AND SCREENS

**Q 5.** **The following statements regarding intensification factor (IF) are true**

**A.** IF is defined as the ratio of − [exposure required for a film + screen] : [exposure required for film alone]

**B.** Typical values for IF are 120–150

**C.** IF decreases when the kV is increased

**D.** IF is increased by using both smaller phosphor crystals and reducing the thickness of the phosphor layer on a screen

**E.** Tungstate screens have a larger IF than rare earth screens

## XERORADIOGRAPHY

**Q 6.** **The following statements are true**

**A.** In mammography, the average dose to glandular tissue in the breast is 2 mGy per mammogram

**B.** In xeroradiography, double-emulsion film in a light-tight cassette is used

**C.** In xeroradiography, the final image is transferred to paper as opposed to film

**D.** Xeroradiography generally incurs a lower dose to the patient than the use of film-screen combinations

**E.** In xeroradiography, the boundaries of a structure are particularly well delineated

## GAMMA IMAGING

**Q 7.** **The following are true**

**A.** 400 mm general purpose gamma camera is optimised for Tc-99 m

**B.** Mobile gamma cameras are designed primarily for renal imaging

**C.** A large field of view camera is used principally for cardiac imaging

**D.** A general-purpose collimator has a resolution of 5 mm

**E.** Low-energy collimators can be used with gamma rays of up to 400 keV

## FILMS AND SCREENS

**Q 8.** **Regarding intensifying screens**

**A.** A phosphorescent film is used

**B.** A reflecting coat of iron oxide is used

**C.** Rare earth phosphors have a higher absorption efficiency compared to calcium tungstate phosphors

**D.** Light-absorbing dyes are used to improve the sharpness of the image

**E.** Light-absorbing dyes are used to minimise the effect of quantum mottle

## X-RAY INTERACTIONS

**Q 9.** **Regarding the interaction of X-rays with matter**

**A.** At 60 keV, the attenuation in fat is predominantly due to Compton interaction

**B.** At 30 keV, attenuation in bone is predominantly due to the photoelectric affect

**C.** In soft tissue, the majority of electrons may be considered as free electrons

**D.** Regarding the Compton effect, the electron density is constant for all elements

**E.** Scatter is more likely to occur in any direction with increase in photon energy

## DOSIMETRY

**Q 10. Regarding the 'air gap' technique**

**A.** An air gap of at least 30 cm is required

**B.** The mAs should be increased

**C.** A screen with a high intensification factor should be used

**D.** The object to film distance is increased

**E.** Scattered radiation travelling obliquely misses the film

## X-RAY TUBES

**Q 11. Regarding X-ray production**

**A.** The filament is raised to incandescence to produce a space charge of protons around the filament by the process of thermionic emission

**B.** Tungsten is used as the filament material because it is relatively inexpensive

**C.** A compound anode is usually made of copper and tin

**D.** The mA is related to the filament current

**E.** X-ray production is over 99% efficient

## IMAGE QUALITY

**Q 12. Secondary radiation grids**

**A.** They absorb only secondary radiation

**B.** The usual range of grid ratio is 4–16

**C.** In general, the higher the lead content of a grid, the more efficient it becomes

**D.** The focal point of a parallel grid is at infinity

**E.** Grid factor is the ratio of incident to transmitted radiation

## FILMS AND SCREENS

**Q 13. Regarding film copying**

**A.** Film copying utilises the principal of solarisation

**B.** With solarisation film, an increase in exposure produces an increase in density

**C.** The theory of solarisation involves the re-bromination hypothesis

**D.** Solarisation emulsion is exposed with a red light source

**E.** Copy film is processed in the same way as standard X-ray film

## GAMMA IMAGING

**Q 14. Comparing the radionuclides krypton-81 m (Kr-81 m) and technetium-99 m (Tc-99 m)**

**A.** Kr-81 m has a longer half-life

**B.** Kr-81 m emits a lower energy gamma ray

**C.** Tc-99 m is less widely used than Kr-81 m

**D.** Tc-99 m has a longer half-life than its parent Mo-99

**E.** Kr-81 m is used for lung ventilation studies

## X-RAY INTERACTIONS

**Q 15. Regarding the photoelectric effect**

**A.** It is the predominant interaction between X-rays and tissues when the photon energy exceeds 60 KeV

**B.** Occurs only when the binding energy of an electron and the photon energy are identical

**C.** May result in the generation of X-rays

**D.** Results in ionisation

**E.** Causes tissue heating in magnetic resonance imaging (MRI), during the application of the radiofrequency pulse

## X-RAY TUBES

**Q 16. Regarding X-ray tubes**

**A.** Rating of a tube is optimised if an exposure occupies less time than 1 revolution of the anode

**B.** The rating of a tube is greater from a 3-phase supply than a half-wave rectified one

**C.** Rotating anode tubes conduct heat as fast as possible via their bearings

**D.** The rating of a tube is increased when a small focal spot is used

**E.** A rotating anode tube cannot be used with a self-rectifying circuit

# FILMS AND SCREENS

**Q 17. The following statements are true**

    **A.** Poor film screen contact increases screen unsharpness

    **B.** Unsharpness due to parallax commonly occurs in single emulsion films

    **C.** Unsharpness due to crossover occurs most commonly in films with tabular grains

    **D.** Single emulsion films are used in nuclear medicine and digital imaging

    **E.** Single emulsion films are used when copying X-rays

# CT

**Q 18. Regarding computed tomography (CT)**

    **A.** The spatial resolution (SR) in CT is better than that in conventional radiography

    **B.** The contrast resolution in CT is better than that in conventional radiography

    **C.** The CT number for air is $-100$

    **D.** The CT number for water is 0

    **E.** The X-ray tube in a CT gantry is mounted with its axis parallel to the slice chosen

# GAMMA IMAGING

**Q 19. Regarding quality assurance (QA) in gamma imaging**

    **A.** Field uniformity is typically 1–2%

    **B.** Cobalt-57 may be used to assess flood field uniformity

    **C.** Intrinsic resolution of a gamma camera can be improved by using a thinner crystal

    **D.** Intrinsic resolution refers to the resolution of the gamma camera plus the collimator

    **E.** System resolution is worsened by scattering of gamma rays within the patient

# RADIATION PROTECTION

**Q 20. Radiation Protection**

    **A.** The effective dose limit for a member of the public is 50 mSv/year

B. Brick walls do not provide any useful shielding against diagnostic X-rays

C. Any individual who wears a film badge/thermoluminescent dosemeter (TLD) should be 'classified'

D. For a given film density, increasing the focus-film distance reduces the skin dose to the patient

E. The dose limit for a member of staff who is pregnant is 13 mSv over the declared term of her pregnancy

## RADIATION PROTECTION

**Q 21. The following are true regarding the Medicines (Administration of Radioactive Substances) Regulations 1978 [M(ARS)R 78]**

A. Administration of radioactive substances should only be carried out by an Administration of Radioactive Substances Advisory Committee ARSAC certificate holder

B. ARSAC certificates are issued by the Department of Health

C. ARSAC certificates are issued to a set group of clinicians within an X-ray department

D. Employers are responsible for the patients treated under the Act

E. An application for an ARSAC certificate must be signed by the radiation protection supervisor

## RADIATION PROTECTION

**Q 22. The following statements regarding doses and dose rates are true**

A. Fluoroscopy – dose rate at the input phosphor: 1 μGy/second

B. Cine-radiography – dose rate at the input prosper: 1 μGy/frame

C. Digital imaging: 1 μGy/frame

D. Photospot film: 10 μGy/frame

E. Skin doses may be up to 300 times greater than the dose to the input phosphor

## RADIATION PROTECTION

**Q 23. The following effective doses are appropriate for the following radiographic procedures**

A. CXR: 0.02 mSv

B. IVU: 2 mSv

**C.** Barium meal: 2 mSv

**D.** Barium enema: 5 mSv

**E.** CT abdomen: 4 mSv

## RADIATION PROTECTION

### Q 24. Radiation protection

**A.** Absorbed dose = energy deposited per unit area

**B.** In most medical applications, the equivalent dose is numerically equal to the absorbed dose in tissues

**C.** The radiation-weighting factor for neutrons and alpha particles is five times greater than that of electrons

**D.** The units of equivalent dose are the Sievert

**E.** The effective dose is the sum of the weighted equivalent doses for all the tissues which have been exposed

## RADIATION PROTECTION

### Q 25. The following statements are true

**A.** If a tube is operated for 1 h, the leakage of radiation at a distance of 1 m from the focus must not total more than 10 mGy

**B.** The housing and support plate of an image intensifier have a lead equivalence of 1.0 mm

**C.** When palpating a patient, a glove of at least 0.25 mm lead equivalence should be worn

**D.** A 0.25 mm lead equivalent body apron typically transmits only 10% of 90 degree scatter

**E.** In interventional radiology, body aprons should have a minimum of 0.35 mm lead equivalence

**A 1.**   **A.** true   **B.** false   **C.** false   **D.** false   **E.** true

The efficiency of production of light in a calcium tungstate screen is only 5%, whereas that in rare earth screens approaches 20%. Lanthanum oxybromide fluoresces blue light.
Intensification factor is the ratio of the exposure needed without screens to exposure needed with the screen.

Armstrong. *Lecture Notes on the Physics of Radiology*, 1st Edn. Clinical Press Ltd., 1990.

**A 2.**   **A.** true   **B.** true   **C.** true   **D.** true   **E.** true

As the images recorded directly from the intensifier output phosphor, there is some loss of information as the film is square and the output phosphor circular. 70 mm cameras are capable of operating at up to 6 frames/second. Due to the short exposure times required a photo-timer is necessary for consistent results.

Armstrong. *Lecture Notes on the Physics of Radiology*, 1st Edn. Clinical Press Ltd., 1990.

**A 3.**   **A.** false   **B.** true   **C.** false   **D.** true   **E.** false

Coherent scattering counts for less than 5% of the interactions in the diagnostic energy range.
In coherent scattering, radiation undergoes a change in direction without a change in wavelength, and therefore no change in energy.

Curry, Thomas. *Christensen's Physics of Diagnostic Radiology,* 4th Edn. Williams & Wilkins (Europe) Ltd.

**A 4.**   **A.** true   **B.** false   **C.** true   **D.** false   **E.** true

As long as the tube KVp is high enough, the majority of interactions occur between filament electrons and K shell electrons of the target material.

The mAs is responsible for the energy of any electrons that make up tube current.

Curry, Thomas. *Christensen's Physics of Diagnostic Radiology*, 4th Edn. Williams & Wilkins (Europe) Ltd.

**A 5.** **A.** false **B.** false **C.** false **D.** false **E.** false

IF = [exposure required for film alone] : [exposure required for the film + screen].
A typical range for IF = 30–100.
IF increases with increasing kV.
IF is increased with larger crystals and increasing thickness of the phosphor layer.
Rare earth screen have a larger IF than tungstate screens.

Farr. Allisy-Roberts. *Physics for Medical Imaging. 1st Edition,* W. B. Saunders Co. Ltd.

**A 6.** **A.** true **B.** false **C.** true **D.** false **E.** true

The average dose of 2 mGy per mammogram carries a risk of inducing a fatal cancer of approximately 20 per million at 30–50 years of age and 10 per million at 50–65 years of age.
In Xeroradiography a sheet of aluminium coated with a layer of selenium is used instead of film. The final image is transferred to paper which is then heated to permanently bond the toner particles.
Xeroradiography generally incurs a higher dose to the patient than the use of film-screen combinations.
This is known as edge enhancement.

Farr, Allisy-Roberts. *Physics for Medical Imaging,* 1st Edn. W. B. Saunders Co. Ltd.

**A 7.** **A.** true **B.** false **C.** false **D.** false **E.** false

Mobile gamma cameras are used in cardiac imaging: 250 mm field and 5 mm thick crystal. This makes it relatively easy to position.
A large field of view camera is used for bone and gallium imaging. These cameras can take in the whole width of a patient.
A general-purpose collimator has a resolution of 9 mm.

Low-energy collimators can be used with gamma rays of up to 150 keV e.g., Tc-99 m.

Farr, Allisy-Roberts. *Physics for Medical Imaging*, 1st Edn. W. B. Saunders Co. Ltd.

**A** **8.**   **A.** false   **B.** false   **C.** true   **D.** true   **E.** false

The phosphors used in intensifying screens are fluorescent.
The reflecting coat is made of a white substance such as titanium oxide.
Light-absorbing dyes help to prevent diffusion of light in the phosphor layer, which acts to reduce the area of the film exposed to light. The screen unsharpness is therefore reduced.
The use of light-absorbing dyes reduces quantum mottle indirectly. This is achieved by the absorption of a greater proportion of the emitted light by the dyes, necessitating a greater exposure. Consequently, quantum mottle also tends to be reduced slightly.

Curry, Thomas. *Christensen's Physics of Diagnostic Radiology*, 4th Edn. Williams & Wilkins (Europe) Ltd.

**A** **9.**   **A.** true   **B.** true   **C.** true   **D.** false   **E.** false

At very low photon energies, however, the photoelectric interaction becomes more predominant.
The electron density of hydrogen is about twice that of all other elements.
With increasing photon energy, scatter is more likely to occur in a forward direction.

Curry, Thomas. *Christensen's Physics of Diagnostic Radiology*, 4th Edn. Williams & Wilkins (Europe) Ltd.

**A** **10.**   **A.** true   **B.** true   **C.** true   **D.** true   **E.** true

With air gaps of less than 30 cm, a high proportion of scattered radiation still reaches the film.
Due to the increased exposure factors required in the air gap technique, a screen with a high intensification factor is required to reduce tube loading.

Curry, Thomas. *Christensen's Physics of Diagnostic Radiology*, 4th Edn. Williams & Wilkins (Europe) Ltd.

A space charge of electrons is produced around the filament. Tungsten is used as the filament material because it is a good thermionic emitter and does not vaporise easily.
A compound anode is usually made of copper and tungsten. X-ray production is less than 1% efficient; the remaining energy is lost as heat.

Curry, Thomas. *Christensen's Physics of Diagnostic Radiology*, 4th Edn. Williams & Wilkins (Europe) Ltd.

**A** **12.** **A.** false   **B.** true   **C.** true   **D.** true   **E.** false

In practice some primary radiation is also absorbed in conjunction with a secondary radiation. As a result, the exposure factors need to be increased when a grid is used.
The ratio of incident to transmitted radiation describes Bucky factor. Grid factor is the ratio of the exposure required with a grid to that without a grid. The usual range is 2–6.

Armstrong. *Lecture Notes on the Physics of Radiology,* 1st Edn. Clinical Press Ltd., 1990.

**A** **13.** **A.** true   **B.** false   **C.** true   **D.** false   **E.** true

Solarisation means that increased exposure actually destroys the developable state. Hence, an increase in exposure produces a decrease in density.
Solarised film is exposed with an ultraviolet light source. Low-density areas in the original X-rays allow more light through and are hence reproduced as areas of low density on the copy film.

Armstrong. *Lecture Notes on the Physics of Radiology,* 1st Edn. Clinical Press Ltd., 1990.

**A** **14.** **A.** false   **B.** false   **C.** false   **D.** false   **E.** true

The half life of Kr-81 m is 13 s compared to the half-life of Tc-99 m of 6h.
Kr-81 m emits a 190-KeV gamma ray, whereas Tc-99 m emits a 140-KeV gamma ray.
Tc-99 m is the main stay radionuclide used in everyday practice.

Exam 2

Answers

Molybdenum-99 has a half-life of 67 h.

Curry, Thomas. *Christensen's Physics of Diagnostic Radiology*, 4th Edn. Williams & Wilkins (Europe) Ltd.

Exam 2

**A** 15.  **A.** false  **B.** false  **C.** true  **D.** true  **E.** false

Photoelectric interactions predominate at low photon energies (e.g., 30 keV). The interaction is proportional to the cube of Z and inversely proportional to the cube of the photon energy.
Photoelectric interactions can only occur if the photon energy applied is greater than the nuclide binding energy of, for example, a K shell electron.
In MRI, the tissue heating during the application of a radiofrequency pulse is due to the electromagnetic energy contained within the radio frequency applied X-rays, and as a consequence their interactions, are not involved in MRI.

Answers

Curry, Thomas. *Christensen's Physics of Diagnostic Radiology*, 4th Edn. Williams & Wilkins (Europe) Ltd.

**A** 16.  **A.** true  **B.** true  **C.** false  **D.** false  **E.** false

Minimal heat is conducted along the anode stem to the bearings. Heat is lost via radiation through the vacuum to the insulating oil. From here it is conducted to the tube housing.
Rating falls with the use of a small focal spot.
A self-rectifying circuit can be used with rotating anodes, but X-rays are only produced during half of the AC voltage supply.

Armstrong. *Lecture Notes on the Physics of Radiology,* 1st Edn. Clinical Press Ltd.

**A** 17.  **A.** true  **B.** false  **C.** false  **D.** true  **E.** true

Parallax is seen with double-emulsion films.
Unsharpness due to crossover commonly occurs with granular/globular grains.

Farr, Allisy-Roberts. *Physics for Medical Imaging*, 1st Edn. W. B. Saunders Co. Ltd.

**A 18.** **A.** false   **B.** true   **C.** false   **D.** true   **E.** false

The SR in CT is only 1 lp/mm, whilst a detailed film-screen combination may have an SR of 10 lp/mm.
The improved contrast resolution of CT is visualised by the use of windowing.
The CT number of air is $-1000$.
The X-ray tube is mounted perpendicular to the slice chosen, in order to reduce any heel effect.

Farr, Allisy-Roberts. *Physics for Medical Imaging*, 1st Edn. W. B. Saunders Co. Ltd.

**A 19.** **A.** true   **B.** true   **C.** true   **D.** false   **E.** true

Intrinsic resolution refers to the resolution of the camera only.
System resolution is the additional blurring caused by the collimator and by scattering within the patient. Consequently, it is worse for fat rather than thin patients.

Farr, Allisy-Roberts. *Physics for Medical Imaging,* 1st Edn. W. B. Saunders Co. Ltd.

**A 20.** **A.** false   **B.** false   **C.** false   **D.** true   **E.** false

The effective dose limit for a member of the public is 1 mSv/year.
120 mm of concrete provides approximately equal protective power against X-rays as 1 mm of lead.
Staff who are likely to exceed 30% of any annual dose limit for workers need to be designated as 'classified'.
Once pregnancy has been declared, the mother should not receive more than 1 mSv to the foetus for the remainder of her pregnancy.

Armstrong. *Lecture Notes on the Physics of Radiology*, 1st Edn. Clinical Press Ltd.

**A 21.** **A.** false   **B.** true   **C.** false   **D.** false   **E.** false

Administration of radioactive substances can be carried out under the clinical supervision of a person holding the ARSAC certificate.
The ARSAC certificate is issued to an individual clinician.
Clinicians are responsible for the patients treated under the Act.

The application for an ARSAC certificate must be signed by a radiation protection advisor.

Farr, Allisy-Roberts. *Physics for Medical Imaging,* 1st Edn. W. B. Saunders Co. Ltd.

**A** **22.** **A.** true   **B.** false   **C.** false   **D.** false   **E.** true

Cine-radiography: 0.1 $\mu$Gy/frame
Digital imaging: 10 $\mu$Gy/frame
Photospot film: 1 $\mu$Gy/frame

Farr, Allisy-Roberts. *Physics for Medical Imaging*, 1st Edn. W. B. Saunders Co. Ltd.

**A** **23.** **A.** true   **B.** false   **C.** false   **D.** false   **E.** false

IVU: 5 mSv.
Ba meal: 5 mSv.
Ba enema: 9 mSv.
CT abdomen: 8 mSv.

Farr, Allisy-Roberts. *Physics for Medical Imaging*, 1st Ed. W. B. Saunders Co. Ltd.

**A** **24.** **A.** false   **B.** true   **C.** false   **D.** true   **E.** true

Absorbed dose = energy deposited per unit mass (J/kg or Gy).
The equivalent dose is numerically equal to the absorbed dose as both X-rays and gamma rays have a radiation-weighting factor of 1.
Neutrons and alpha particles have a radiation-weighting factor 10–20 times greater than that of electrons.
One Sv = J/kg.

Farr, Allisy-Roberts. *Physics for Medical Imaging,* 1st Edn. W. B. Saunders Co. Ltd.

**A** **25.** **A.** false   **B.** false   **C.** true   **D.** true   **E.** true

The maximum permitted leakage is 1 mGy.
The housing and support plate have a lead equivalence of 2.5 mm.

Farr, Allisy-Roberts. *Physics for Medical Imaging*, 1st Edn. W. B. Saunders Co. Ltd.

# Questions

## FILMS AND SCREENS

**Q 1. The following types of screen can be used with film sensitive to the blue region of the light spectrum**

- **A.** Calcium tungstate screens
- **B.** Barium strontium sulphate screens
- **C.** Silver-activated zinc sulphide screens
- **D.** Zinc cadmium sulphide (ZnCdS) screens
- **E.** Terbium-activated screens

## X-RAY INTERACTIONS

**Q 2. The amount of scatter reaching the film may be reduced by**

- **A.** Restricting field size
- **B.** Decreasing the part thickness irradiated
- **C.** Using an air gap technique
- **D.** Using a secondary radiation grid
- **E.** Placing a filter between the X-ray tube and the patient

## X-RAY TUBES

**Q 3. Regarding the focal spot**

- **A.** Focal spot size decreases with an increase in the tube current
- **B.** Focal spot size increases with an increase in kVp
- **C.** The modulation transfer function (MTF) worsens with an increase in the focal spot size
- **D.** A star test pattern-imaging tool is useful for assessing focal spot sizes of less than 0.3 mm
- **E.** The star test pattern measures the actual focal spot size

# DOSIMETRY

### Q 4.  Regarding the Geiger-Muller (GM) tube

A.  The outer cylinder is the anode
B.  Detection of ionising radiation occurs through the process of gas amplification
C.  The anode and the cathode are surrounded by hydrogen gas
D.  The tube is sensitive to the detection of high-energy radiation
E.  A voltage of 25 kV is applied across the tube

# IMAGE QUALITY

### Q 5.  Regarding resolution of an image

A.  Resolution may be expressed as line pairs per mm
B.  Line spread function (LSF) is calculated from an image produced by a narrow line source of X-rays
C.  When measuring LSF, image boundaries are less well recorded with high-speed screens than with slower-speed screens
D.  The LSF of an X-ray exposed without a screen deteriorates as compared to a film exposed with a screen
E.  The resolving power of an imaging system is its ability to record, as separate images, small objects placed very close together

# RADIOACTIVITY

### Q 6.  Regarding radioactivity

A.  Is a random process
B.  Is produced when annihilation radiation is produced
C.  Is an exponential decay process for a given radionuclide
D.  Is more likely to happen when a radioactive source is heated
E.  Beta particles have a range of only a few millimetres

# GAMMA IMAGING

### Q 7.  Regarding a photomultiplier tube

A.  Electrons are accelerated through a series of dynodes
B.  It needs to be shielded from light

C. The insides of the tube are coated with a reflective layer
D. The tube contains a vacuum
E. Radiations of different energies can be distinguished from each other

## X-RAY INTERACTIONS

**Q 8.   Regarding the mass attenuation coefficient (MAC)**

A. Of an absorber, is proportional to the linear attenuation co-efficient of the absorber
B. Of water is greater than that of ice
C. Of an absorber, varies with the physical density of that absorber
D. Has units of grams per square centimetre
E. Is equal to the density of an absorber divided by its linear attenuation coefficient

## X-RAY TUBES

**Q 9.   X-ray production**

A. In all forms of diagnostic radiology, 80% or more of the X-rays emitted are Bremsstrahlung radiation
B. The photon energy of the K-radiation increases as the atomic number of the target increases
C. Increasing the kV shifts the X-ray spectrum curve to the left
D. Increasing the mA does not affect the shape of the X-ray spectrum
E. The ripple factor for a 6-phase generator is less than that of a 12-phase generator

## IMAGE QUALITY

**Q 10.   Secondary radiation grids**

A. The line density of a moving grid is typically 25 lines/mm
B. Grid lines reduce fine detail definition on an X-ray
C. Crossed grids are more efficient at removing scattered radiation than uncrossed grids
D. Decreased exposure doses are required when using a crossed grid as opposed to an uncrossed grid
E. Moiré fringes are typically seen with uncrossed grids

# FILMS AND SCREENS

### Q 11. Regarding films and screens

A. The front of an X-ray cassette is usually made of aluminium or carbon fibre

B. The back of an X-ray cassette usually incorporates a thin lead sheet to reduce backscatter

C. An intensifying screen consists of a polyester base 0.25 mm thick with phosphor crystals 3–10 μ in size

D. The most frequently used phosphors in an intensifying screen are calcium tungstate, lanthanum and gadolinium

E. Rare earths screens are more efficient than tungsten in converting absorbed X-rays into light

# FILMS AND SCREENS

### Q 12. Exposure factors

A. A high mAs is generally desirable when selecting exposure factors

B. The kV chosen should be as high as possible when selecting exposure factors

C. Exposure times can be reduced by using a larger focal spot

D. Exposure times can be reduced by using a single-phase generator rather than a three-phase generator

E. Exposure times can be reduced by using both a lower speed and smaller diameter anode disc

# GAMMA IMAGING

### Q 13. Regarding the gamma camera

A. Sensitivity can be measured by imaging a line source

B. The use of a thinner crystal improves sensitivity

C. Quantum mottle is improved by using a shorter exposure

D. Spatial resolution is unaffected by high count rates

E. Gamma imaging is said to be 'noise limited'

# FILMS AND SCREENS

**Q 14.  Regarding unsharpness**

    **A.**  Parallax unsharpness is usually seen when viewing wet film

    **B.**  In order to minimise total unsharpness, the values of the separate unsharpness components should approximate each other

    **C.**  Screen unsharpness results from diffusion of light within the screen phosphor

    **D.**  Poor film screen contact increases the degree of unsharpness

    **E.**  Fast screens have an unsharpness of about 0.3 mm

# X-RAY INTERACTIONS AND FILTERS

**Q 15.  The air gap technique**

    **A.**  There is a significant degree of filtration within the air gap itself

    **B.**  In the diagnostic energy range there is a strong bias towards forward scattering

    **C.**  The results are equivalent to using a grid, but higher patient exposures are necessary

    **D.**  In order to preserve image sharpness, the focus to film distance needs to be increased in conjunction with an increase in object to film distance

    **E.**  The ratio of scattered to primary radiation reaching the film for a given thickness of an absorber depends on the size of the air gap present

# X-RAY TUBES

**Q 16.  Regarding X-ray generating apparatus**

    **A.**  In the transformer assembly the filament circuit is supplied by a step-down transformer

    **B.**  In the transformer assembly the potential difference across the step-up transformer is usually 50 kV

    **C.**  The transformer assembly contains oil which acts to prevent electrical sparking between the transformer assembly components

**D.** In the filament circuit a potential difference of about 100 V is applied across the filament

**E.** In the filament circuit a current of 3–5 A is usually produced through the filament

## TOMOGRAPHY

Q 17. **The following are true regarding tomography**

   **A.** In autotomography the X-ray tube moves in a circular arc

   **B.** In autotomography exposure times in the order of 250 ms are used

   **C.** Pantomography is a technique which produces a panoramic radiograph of a curved surface

   **D.** In pantomography both the X-ray tube and film rotate during an exposure

   **E.** In orthopantomography (OPG) the X-ray apparatus changes its axis of rotation twice during a single exposure

## IMAGE QUALITY

Q 18. **Regarding grids used in radiography**

   **A.** They improve contrast

   **B.** The grid ratio is defined as the ratio of total area covered by the lead foil strips to the total area covered by the interspace material

   **C.** Consists of a series of lead strips separated by a transparent spacing material

   **D.** The grid ratio for a crossed grid is equal to the product of the ratios of the two superimposed linear grids

   **E.** An X-ray tube can be angled when using a linear grid without cut-off occurring

## GAMMA IMAGING

Q 19. **Gamma imaging**

   **A.** Rectilinear scanners produce images more slowly than gamma cameras

   **B.** A high-energy collimator is routinely used when imaging with Technetium-99 m

   **C.** Radioisotopes are less well resolved at depth in tissue compared to those near the skin

**D.** A desirable isotope should have a short half-life to reduce patient dose

**E.** The greater the sensitivity of a collimator, the lower its spatial resolution

## RADIATION PROTECTION

Q 20. **The following statements are true**

**A.** Local rules are enforced by the radiation protection supervisor (RPS)

**B.** Local rules are a legal document

**C.** The department of the environment is responsible for enforcing the Radioactive Substances Act 1993

**D.** The Health & Safety Executive (HSE) is responsible for enforcing the Ionising Radiations Regulations 1999 (IRR 99)

**E.** The Department of the Environment is responsible for enforcing the IRR 99

## RADIATION PROTECTION

Q 21. **The following are true**

**A.** Increasing kV reduces the skin dose to the patient

**B.** Increasing kV reduces the dose to deeper tissues

**C.** Increasing the focus to film distance (FFD) reduces patient dose

**D.** The entrance dose for a PA chest X-ray is greater than that of an AP abdominal X-ray

**E.** Skin dose increases exponentially with increasing mAs

## RADIATION PROTECTION

Q 22. **The following statements are true**

**A.** Human error resulting in serious patient over-exposure should be investigated by the Department of Health (DoH)

**B.** Equipment fault causing a patient over-exposure greater than twice the dose intended, results in the equipment being withdrawn from use

**C.** The Department of Health should always be informed of equipment failures

**D.** It is not necessary to retain the completed request form after an X-ray has been taken

**E.** The Department of Health recommends that films and other records be kept for a minimum of 6 years

## RADIATION PROTECTION

**Q** **23. Regarding radionuclides and their effective doses**

**A.** Tc-99 m macroaggregates (MAA) of albumin: effective dose (ED) = 5 mSv

**B.** Galium-67: ED = 18 mSv

**C.** Tc-99 m MAG3: ED = 1 mSv

**D.** Kr-81 m gas: ED = 1 mSv

**E.** Tc-99 m phosphonates: ED = 1 mSv

## RADIATION PROTECTION

**Q** **24. The following entrance doses are appropriate for the following radiographs**

**A.** AP lumbar spine X-ray: 10 mGy

**B.** AP abdominal X-ray: 5 mGy

**C.** AP pelvic X-ray: 5 mGy

**D.** PA chest X-ray: 0.3 mGy

**E.** PA skull X-ray: 5 mGy

## RADIATION PROTECTION

**Q** **25. Persons may receive higher radiation doses in the following types of work**

**A.** Cardiac catheterisation

**B.** Interventional radiology

**C.** Radiopharmaceutical preparation

**D.** Nursing a patient undergoing brachytherapy

**E.** Preparation and insertion of radioactive implants

**A 1.** **A.** true **B.** true **C.** true **D.** false **E.** false

The light emission from calcium tungstate, barium strontium sulphate and silver-activated zinc sulphide screens occurs in the blue region of the light spectrum.
ZnCdS is used as the output phosphor in an image intensifier. It emits light in the yellow-green region.
Terbium is an activator in rarer screens which emit light in the yellow-green region.

Curry, Thomas. *Christensen's Physics of Diagnostic Radiology,* 4th Edn. Williams & Wilkins (Europe) Ltd.

**A 2.** **A.** true **B.** true **C.** true **D.** true **E.** false

A filter in this position removes the useless low-energy radiation which would not have had sufficient energy to reach the film.

Curry, Thomas. *Christensen's Physics of Diagnostic Radiology,* 4th Edn. Williams & Wilkins (Europe) Ltd.

**A 3.** **A.** false **B.** false **C.** true **D.** true **E.** false

Focal spot size increases with an increase in the tube current. This effect is called 'blooming' and is more marked at low peak kVp and high mAs.
The focal spot size decreases slightly with increasing peak kVp.
The pinhole camera technique measures actual focal spot size, whereas the star test pattern measures the resolving capacity of the focal spot.

Curry, Thomas. *Christensen's Physics of Diagnostic Radiology*, 4th Edn. Williams & Wilkins (Europe) Ltd.

**A 4.** **A.** false **B.** true **C.** false **D.** false **E.** false

The outer case is the cathode.
The tube is usually surrounded by an inert gas, usually argon, which is combined with either alcohol vapour or a halogen gas, and maintained at low atmospheric pressure (10 cmHg).
High-energy radiation tends to pass through the tube and is thus less likely to be detected.
A voltage of 900–1,050 V is applied across the tube when alcohol vapour is used. Alternatively a voltage of 200–400 V is applied when a halogen gas is used.

Curry, Thomas. *Christensen's Physics of Diagnostic Radiology*, 4th Edn. Williams & Wilkins (Europe) Ltd.

**A 5.** **A.** true **B.** true **C.** true **D.** false **E.** true

The LSF of an X-ray film which is exposed without screens is improved, as there is no light diffusion from the screen.

Armstrong. *Lecture Notes on the Physics of Radiology*, 1st Edn. Clinical Press Ltd., 1990.

**A 6.** **A.** true **B.** false **C.** true **D.** false **E.** true

When a positron and an electron annihilate each other, electromagnetic radiation is emitted.
The process of radioactivity is not influenced by external factors.

Curry, Thomas. *Christensen's Physics of Diagnostic Radiology*, 4th Edn. Williams & Wilkins (Europe) Ltd.

**A 7.** **A.** true **B.** true **C.** true **D.** true **E.** true

If external light were not excluded, incident light would stimulate the photocathode and produce a pulse. The inside is coated to reflect back any light that might otherwise have escaped. Different energies can be assessed, as the size of the electrical pulse emitted is proportional to the amount of light emitted from the photocathode. This in turn is proportional to the energy of the incident photon. The dynodes act as an amplification process for the photoelectrons emitted, so as to produce a readable output current from the tube.

Curry, Thomas. *Christensen's Physics of Diagnostic Radiology*, 4th Edn. Williams & Wilkins (Europe) Ltd.

**A 8.** **A.** true   **B.** false   **C.** false   **D.** false   **E.** false

The MAC of water is identical to that of ice.
The MAC is independent of the physical density of an absorber.
MAC has units of square cm per gram.
The MAC equals the linear attenuation coefficient (LAC) divided by the physical density of an absorber.

Curry, Thomas. *Christensen's Physics of Diagnostic Radiology*, 4th Edn. Williams & Wilkins (Europe) Ltd.

**A 9.** **A.** false   **B.** true   **C.** false   **D.** true   **E.** false

In mammography, characteristic radiation forms the majority of the X-ray spectrum.
Increasing the kV shifts the X-ray spectrum curve to the right.
Increasing mAs increases tube output.
Ripple factor: 6-phase generator –13%; 12-phase generator – 3%

Farr, Allisy-Roberts. *Physics for Medical Imaging*, 1st Edn. W. B. Saunders Co. Ltd.

**A 10.** **A.** false   **B.** true   **C.** true   **D.** false   **E.** false

Line density of a moving grid = 5 lines/mm
Increased exposure doses and careful centring are required with crossed grids.
Moiré fringes are a coarse interference pattern seen when the crossed grids are not at right angles to each other.

Farr, Allisy-Roberts. *Physics for Medical Imaging*, 1st Edn. W. B. Saunders Co. Ltd.

**A 11.** **A.** true   **B.** true   **C.** true   **D.** true   **E.** true

Aluminium and carbon fibre reduce attenuation of an X-ray beam, thus reducing patient exposure.

Lanthanum and gadolinium are classed as rare earth phosphors. Rare earth screens are 20% efficient; calcium tungstate screens have an efficiency of 5%.

Farr, Allisy-Roberts. *Physics for Medical Imaging*, 1st Edn. W. B. Saunders Co. Ltd.

A **12.** **A.** false   **B.** true   **C.** true   **D.** false   **E.** false

The mAs should be kept as low as is needed in order to reduce exposure times.
Increasing kV increases penetration and latitude of exposure. However, the kV should not be so high that insufficient contrast results.
Exposure times are reduced by using a three-phase generator rather than a single-phase generator.
Exposure times can be reduced by using a higher speed and larger diameter anode disc.

Farr, Allisy-Roberts. *Physics for Medical Imaging*, 1st Edn. W. B. Saunders Co. Ltd.

A **13.** **A.** false   **B.** false   **C.** false   **D.** false   **E.** true

Sensitivity is assessed by imaging a flood field phantom.
Using a thinner crystal improves resolution at the expense of decreased sensitivity.
With shorter exposures, counts fluctuate from pixel to pixel resulting in increased noise.
At high count rates, there are an increasing number of counts lost due to the 'dead time' with a consequent reduction in spatial resolution.

Farr, Allisy-Roberts. *Physics for Medical Imaging*, 1st Edn. W. B. Saunders Co. Ltd.

A **14.** **A.** true   **B.** true   **C.** true   **D.** true   **E.** true

Curry, Thomas. *Christensen's Physics of Diagnostic Radiology*, 4th Edn. Williams & Wilkins (Europe) Ltd.

A **15.** **A.** false   **B.** false   **C.** false   **D.** true   **E.** true

The air gap technique is effective because scattered photons simply 'miss' the film.

No forward scattering bias exists. In the diagnostic energy range a photon is likely to be scattered equally in any direction.
Lower patient exposures are necessary than with a grid.
A large air gap will reduce the ratio of scattered to primary radiation reaching the film.

Curry, Thomas. *Christensen's Physics of Diagnostic Radiology*, 4th Edn. Williams & Wilkins (Europe) Ltd.

**A** **16. A.** true   **B.** false   **C.** true   **D.** false   **E.** true

The potential difference across the step-up transformer may be as much as 150 kV.
In the filament circuit, an incoming mains supply of 220 V is stepped-down to provide a potential difference of about 10 V across the filament.

Armstrong. *Lecture Notes on the Physics of Radiology*, 1st Edn. Clinical Press Ltd., 1990.

**A** **17. A.** false   **B.** false   **C.** true   **D.** true   **E.** true

Autotomography is a technique which involves patient movement while keeping the X-ray tube and film stationary. Long exposure times, in the order of 5 s, are used for this technique.
The OPG machine needs to change its axis of rotation twice to allow for angulation of the jaw.

Armstrong. *Lecture Notes on the Physics of Radiology*, 1st Edn. Clinical Press Ltd., 1990.

**A** **18. A.** true   **B.** false   **C.** true   **D.** false   **E.** true

The grid ratio is defined as a ratio of the height of the lead strips to the distance between them.
The grid ratio of a crossed grid is equal to the sum of the two superimposed linear grids.

Armstrong. *Lecture Notes on the Physics of Radiology*, 1st Edn. Clinical Press Ltd.

**A** 19. **A.** true  **B.** false  **C.** true  **D.** true  **E.** true

Tc-99 m emits a gamma ray of 140 KeV. This is usually used in conjunction with a low-energy general-purpose collimator.

Curry, Thomas. *Christensen's Physics of Diagnostic Radiology,* 4th Edn. Williams & Wilkins (Europe) Ltd.

**A** 20. **A.** false  **B.** true  **C.** true  **D.** true  **E.** false

The local rules are policed by the RPS, but enforced by the local HSE Inspector.
Enforcing the IRR 99 is the responsibility of the Secretary of State for Health who uses the appropriate HSE.

Farr, Allisy-Roberts. *Physics for Medical Imaging*, 1st Edn. W. B. Saunders Co. Ltd.

**A** 21. **A.** true  **B.** true  **C.** true  **D.** false  **E.** false

The entrance dose for a PA chest X-ray = 0.3 mGy: AP abdomen = 10 mGy.
Skin dose increases linearly with increasing mAs.

Farr, Allisy-Roberts. *Physics for Medical Imaging*, 1st Edn. W. B. Saunders Co. Ltd.

**A** 22. **A.** true  **B.** false  **C.** true  **D.** false  **E.** true

If the over-exposure is greater than 3 times the dose intended, the equipment should be withdrawn. Nevertheless, all faults should be investigated and rectified.
The DoH should always be informed so that hazard-warning notices can be issued nationally as appropriate.
A completed request form, signed by a medical practitioner, is a legal document and should be retained, often in the X-ray packet.
Films and records should be kept for 6 years for possible future litigation and for calculations of total patient dose.

Farr, Allisy-Roberts. *Physics for Medical Imaging*, 1st Edn. W. B. Saunders Co. Ltd.

**A** 23. **A.** false  **B.** true  **C.** true  **D.** false  **E.** false

Tc-99m MAA: ED – 1 mSv.
Kr-81m: ED – 0.1 mSv.
Tc-99m phosphonates: ED – 5 mSv.

Farr, Allisy-Roberts. *Physics for Medical Imaging*, 1st Edn. W. B. Saunders Co. Ltd.

**A** 24. **A.** true  **B.** false  **C.** false  **D.** true  **E.** true

AP abdomen: 10 mGy.
AP pelvis: 10 mGy.

Farr, Allisy-Roberts. *Physics for Medical Imaging*, 1st Edn. W. B. Saunders Co. Ltd.

**A** 25. **A.** true  **B.** true  **C.** true  **D.** true  **E.** true

It is unlikely that many persons in a hospital will need to be designated as classified persons on the basis of likely exposure. However, in the types of work listed, persons may receive higher doses.

*Regulation 9 AC1/64. The Ionising Radiations Regulations 1988 (IRR 88).*

# RADIOACTIVITY

**Q 1.  The following are true**

   **A.** The nucleus of an element is composed of neutrons and electrons
   **B.** The half-life of a radioisotope is analogous to the decay constant
   **C.** Beta particles tend to be emitted from nuclides with an excess of electrons
   **D.** When a radioisotope emits a positron, its atomic number decreases by unity
   **E.** A radioisotope in a metastable state emits a gamma ray and turns into another element

# X-RAY INTERACTIONS

**Q 2.  The following are true**

   **A.** Attenuation = absorption − scatter
   **B.** Coherent scattering accounts for generally less than 5% of all X-ray interactions
   **C.** The photoelectric effect results in ionisation of an atom
   **D.** For pair production to occur, the incident radiation must have a minimum energy of at least 1.02 MeV
   **E.** Attenuation of polychromatic radiation is usually exponential

# IMAGE QUALITY

**Q 3.  The following are true:**

   **A.** Magnification is reduced by using a shorter focus to film distance (FFD) or by increasing the object to film distance (OFD)
   **B.** Distortion is increased by using a longer FFD
   **C.** Geometric unsharpness is reduced by using a smaller focal spot

**D.** Geometric unsharpness is increased by increasing the OFD

**E.** Movement unsharpness may be reduced by immobilisation

## X-RAY TUBES

**Q 4.** **Regarding rotating anode tubes (RAT)**

**A.** RATs cool by conduction of heat along the anode stem

**B.** RATs have a limited use in diagnostic radiology

**C.** In routine diagnostic radiology RATs rotate at approximately 15,000 rpm

**D.** The target anode disc is usually made from pure tungsten alone

**E.** Heat dissipation from the anode assembly is proportional to the fourth power of the Kelvin temperature of the anode

## FILMS AND SCREENS

**Q 5.** **The following are true**

**A.** Photographic emulsion is a suspension in gelatin of 50% iodide and 50% bromide

**B.** Photographic emulsion is not affected by creasing or mechanical pressure

**C.** In silver halide crystals, sensitivity specks absorb electrons to form a latent image

**D.** About 90% of X-rays falling on a film cassette are absorbed by the front intensifying screen

**E.** Silver halide crystals are about 1 $\mu$m in size

## FILMS AND SCREENS

**Q 6.** **The following statements are true**

**A.** Automatic exposure control (AEC) cannot be performed with a plate ionisation chamber

**B.** AEC may be carried out using a phosphor coupled to a photomultiplier tube

**C.** AEC devises are generally larger than the film cassette

**D.** When measuring the kV for quality assurance, the actual tube kV should be within $+/-5\%$ of the set value

**E.** A penetrameter is not a suitable method for measuring tube kV

# GAMMA IMAGING

**Q 7.** **Regarding radionuclides**

A. An ideal radionuclide should be polyenergetic
B. An ideal radionuclide should emit both beta particles and gamma rays
C. In a technetium (Tc) generator, at transient equilibrium, Tc-99 m decays with a half-life of 6 h.
D. In a Tc generator, Mo-99 is absorbed onto an alumina exchange column
E. Tc-99 m is eluted with sterile dextrose saline solution

# FILMS AND SCREENS

**Q 8.** **The following are true of X-ray film**

A. In an unexposed film, base plus fog is approximately 0.5
B. Film fogging is independent of the film age
C. Film fogging is independent of the processor temperature
D. The greater the film latitude the lower the film gamma
E. The greater the film latitude the higher the film gamma

# X-RAY TUBES

**Q 9.** **Regarding rectification**

A. Rectification refers to the process of changing direct current into alternating current
B. Full-wave rectification utilises the full potential of the electrical supply in the production of X-rays
C. In a three-phase generator, three separate voltage pulses in phase with each other are produced to provide almost constant potential
D. The ripple factor for a six-pulse generator is 13%
E. The ripple factor for a single-phase generator is 3%

# X-RAY INTERACTIONS

**Q 10.** **The following are ways in which X-ray interact with matter**

A. Coherent scattering
B. Photoelectric effect
C. Compton scattering

**D.** Pair production

**E.** Photodisintegration

# DOSIMETRY

**Q 11. The following are methods of dosimetry**

    **A.** Erythema test dose

    **B.** Conversion of ferric sulphate to ferrous sulphate

    **C.** A colour change induced in barium platinocyanide

    **D.** Change in the colour of litmus paper from blue to red

    **E.** Fluorescence

# XERORADIOGRAPHY

**Q 12. The following are true of xeroradiography**

    **A.** There is better edge contrast

    **B.** Developing speed of a xeroradiographic plate is longer than conventional techniques

    **C.** The dose incurred to the patient is generally higher than film screen systems

    **D.** Special handling is required for the plates

    **E.** The resolution achieved with this technique is relatively poor

# IMAGE QUALITY

**Q 13. The following are true**

    **A.** In a tomogram the contrast is independent of the thickness of the cut

    **B.** The shadow of a circular object held parallel to a film is also circular

    **C.** Magnification is increased when the focus to object distance is increased

    **D.** Radiographic contrast is D2 − D1, where D2 and D1 are optical density on two adjacent areas of a film

    **E.** Contrast depends upon both the thickness and the difference in attenuation coefficients in the structures that go to create it

# RADIATION PHYSICS

**Q 14. Electromagnetic radiation (EMR)**

    **A.** The velocity of EMR in air is about half of that in a vacuum

    **B.** In air, all forms of EMR obeys the inverse square law

C. The wavelength and frequency of EMR are always inversely proportional to each other

D. The intensity of EMR is the amount of energy passing through a unit area per unit time

E. X-rays and gamma rays are of lower photon energy than visible light

## X-RAY INTERACTIONS AND FILTRATION

Q 15. **Regarding filtration**

A. In a compound filter, the higher atomic number material should face the patient

B. Aluminium and tin are the most commonly used compound filters

C. Filters used in diagnostic radiology, reduce the exposure dose to a patient

D. Filtration increases both the minimum and effective photon energies of an X-ray spectrum

E. Excess filtration increases exposure times

## X-RAY TUBES

Q 16. **The following are true**

A. The heel effect is most prominent at the cathode end of the tube

B. The steeper the target the greater the heel effect

C. The shorter the focus to film distance (FFD), the less is the heel effect for a given film size

D. When a body part of considerable varying thickness is to be X-rayed, it is advantageous to place the thicker part towards the cathode side of the tube

E. The intensity of an X-ray beam is uniform across its field

## FILMS AND SCREENS

Q 17. **The following are true**

A. Optical density depends upon the number of silver grains per unit area of film

B. Optical density = Log to base 10 (transmitted light : incident light)

**C.** A logarithmic scale is used for optical density primarily in order to make graphical analysis easier

**D.** If 1% of light from a viewing box is transmitted through an X-ray film, then the optical density is 2.0

**E.** If both the front and rear emulsions of an X-ray film each provide an optical density of 1.2, then the total optical density is equal to the product of these values = 1.44

# IMAGE QUALITY

**Q 18. The following statements are true**

**A.** Focal spot modulation transfer function (MTF) is reduced with macro-radiography

**B.** Screen MTF is increased with macro-radiography

**C.** In macro-radiography, screen unsharpness is also magnified

**D.** In mammography, subject contrast is achieved primarily via photoelectric absorption

**E.** In mammography, an appropriate operating kVp would be 28 kV

# CT

**Q 19. Regarding noise in computed tomography (CT)**

**A.** Noise may be reduced by decreasing the number of photons absorbed in each voxel

**B.** Noise may be reduced by either decreasing slice thickness or reducing pixel size

**C.** Noise may be reduced by either increasing mA or increasing the scan time

**D.** Narrow windowing makes noise more noticeable

**E.** Zoom enlargement of a CT display increases noise

# RADIATION PROTECTION

**Q 20. The following statements are true**

**A.** Any individual is allowed to be present in an X-ray room when radiation is being generated

**B.** The doors of an X-ray room should be closed during examinations

**C.** For persons of reproductive capacity, gonad shields must always be used

**D.** An anteroposterior rather than a posteroanterior, projection of the chest can greatly reduce the dose to the breast

**E.** Phantoms should be used for training in radiography and research into examination techniques

## RADIATION PROTECTION

Q 21. **The following statements are true**

**A.** A dose of 1 Sv to the testes produces sterility
**B.** Non-stochastic effects are threshold dependent
**C.** Stochastic effects are threshold dependent
**D.** A dose of 2 Sv to the eyes will produce cataracts
**E.** A whole body dose of 10 Sv or more is 100% lethal to humans

## RADIATION PROTECTION

Q 22. **Regarding film badge dosimetry**

**A.** Personal monitoring film is exposed with a single intensifying screen
**B.** Personal monitoring film badges are double-coated; one emulsion is slow, the other emulsion is fast
**C.** A film badge contains at least 3 pairs of filters
**D.** Spots of intense blackening seen on a personal monitoring film badge, suggests exposure to high-energy photons
**E.** A single exposure to direct X-rays from one direction, would produce a sharp edge to the shadow of a film badge filter

## RADIATION PROTECTION

Q 23. **The following statements are true**

**A.** Body aprons should be available with a protective equivalent of not less than 0.25 mm lead for X-rays over 100 kV
**B.** Gloves and aprons should be thoroughly examined at least once a month to ensure that no cracks have developed
**C.** During operation of a CT scanner, an operator should be present at the control panel while high voltage is applied to the X-ray tube
**D.** Gloves should be available with protective equivalent of not less than 0.35 mm lead for X-rays up to 150 kV
**E.** Body aprons should not be folded

# RADIATION PROTECTION

**Q** **24. The following statements are true**

    **A.** The annual background radiation exposure per caput of the UK population is about 1.5 mSv

    **B.** Natural radiation contributes 60% of the total per caput radiation exposure from all radiation sources

    **C.** The largest contributor to natural background radiation is from gamma ray exposure

    **D.** Medical exposure contributes approximately 13% of the total per caput radiation exposure from all radiation sources

    **E.** Food and drink contributes approximately 5% of the total per caput radiation exposure from all radiation sources

# RADIATION PROTECTION

**Q** **25. Regarding the Geiger-Muller (GM) tube**

    **A.** It is able to detect any type of ionising radiation

    **B.** It is able to distinguish between different types of radiation and different energies of the same radiation

    **C.** It is more efficient in detecting lower energy as opposed to higher energy beta particles

    **D.** The efficiency of detection for gamma rays is only 10%

    **E.** The principle use is one of contamination monitoring

**A 1.**  **A.** false  **B.** false  **C.** false  **D.** true  **E.** false

The nucleus is composed of protons and neutrons.
The half-life of an isotope is the time taken for the amount of
the radioactivity present to decay to 50% of its original value.
Beta particles tend to be emitted from nuclides with an excess of
neutrons.
A metastable isotope emits a gamma ray and becomes the stable
daughter product of the same element.

Armstrong. *Lecture Notes on the Physics of Radiology*, 1st Edn. Clinical Press
Ltd.

**A 2.**  **A.** false  **B.** true  **C.** true  **D.** true  **E.** false

Attenuation = absorption + scatter.
Attenuation of monochromatic radiation is exponential.

Farr, Allisy-Roberts. *Physics for Medical Imaging*, 1st Edn. W. B. Saunders Co.
Ltd.

**A 3.**  **A.** false  **B.** false  **C.** true  **D.** true  **E.** true

Magnification is reduced by increasing the FFD or decreasing the
OFD.
Distortion is increased when using a shorter FFD.

Farr, Allisy-Roberts. *Physics for Medical Imaging*, 1st Edn. W. B. Saunders Co.
Ltd.

**A 4.**  **A.** false  **B.** false  **C.** false  **D.** false  **E.** true

Cooling is via radiation of heat to the insulating oil and then
conduction to the tube housing.
RATs are widely used in diagnostic radiology.
RATs usually rotate at about 3,000 rpm. High-speed RATs
e.g., 15,000 rpm are used in angiography.

The target is usually tungsten with about 10% rhenium. This has better thermal properties and is less likely to roughen with use.

Farr, Allisy-Roberts. *Physics for Medical Imaging*, 1st Edn. W. B. Saunders Co. Ltd.

**A 5.** **A.** false **B.** false **C.** true **D.** false **E.** true

Photographic emulsion consists of about 90% bromide and 10% iodide.
Emulsion is also affected by chemical liquids and static electricity, which all have implications for storage.
About a third of the X-rays are absorbed by the front screen.

Farr, Allisy-Roberts. *Physics for Medical Imaging*, 1st Edn. W. B. Saunders Co. Ltd.

**A 6.** **A.** false **B.** true **C.** true **D.** true **E.** false

The tube kV may be estimated indirectly by the penetrameter method.

Farr, Allisy-Roberts. *Physics for Medical Imaging*, 1st Edn. W. B. Saunders Co. Ltd.

**A 7.** **A.** false **B.** false **C.** false **D.** true **E.** false

An ideal radionuclide should be monoenergetic, so that scatter can be easily eliminated by the pulse height analyser.
An ideal radionuclide should emit gamma rays only; these produce the image. Beta (and alpha) particles contribute only to patient dose.
At transient equilibrium, both the 'parent' Mo-99 and the 'daughter' Tc-99 m decay together with the half-life of the parent – 67 h.
Tc-99 m is eluted with a sterile saline solute.

Farr, Allisy-Roberts. *Physics for Medical Imaging*, 1st Edn. W. B. Saunders Co. Ltd.

**A 8.** **A.** false **B.** false **C.** false **D.** true **E.** false

Base plus fog is approximately 0.2.
Fogging is increased with both the age of the film and with an increase in processor temperature.

Curry, Thomas. *Christensen's Physics of Diagnostic Radiology*, 4th Edn. Williams & Wilkins (Europe) Ltd.

A 9. **A.** false **B.** true **C.** false **D.** true **E.** false

Rectification refers to the process of changing alternating current into direct current.

Three-phase generators produce three separate voltages which are 120 degrees out of phase with each other to produce almost constant potential.

The variation in the voltage across an X-ray tube expressed as a percentage of the maximum value is the ripple factor. For a six-pulse generator this is 13%, and for a twelve-pulse generator 3%. Single-phase generators have a ripple factor of 100%.

Armstrong. *Lecture Notes on the Physics of Radiology*, 1st Edn. Clinical Press Ltd., 1990.

A 10. **A.** true **B.** true **C.** true **D.** true **E.** true

Armstrong. *Lecture Notes on the Physics of Radiology*, 1st Edn. Clinical Press Ltd., 1990.

A 11. **A.** true **B.** true **C.** true **D.** false **E.** true

Litmus paper is used in the detection of acid or alkali and is not a method of dosimetry.

Armstrong. *Lecture Notes on the Physics of Radiology*, 1st Edn. Clinical Press Ltd., 1990.

A 12. **A.** true **B.** false **C.** true **D.** true **E.** false

As it is possible to use high kVs, with associated less tissue absorption, there is still better edge contrast than with conventional techniques.

There is approximately 30 second development which is dry as no chemicals are involved.

A high resolution is obtained with this technique.

Armstrong. *Lecture Notes on the Physics of Radiology*, 1st Edn. Clinical Press Ltd., 1990.

Exam 4

Answers

**A 13. A.** false **B.** true **C.** false **D.** true **E.** true

In tomography contrast is diminished with the very thin cuts. Magnification is the ratio of the focus-film distance (FFD) to focus-object distance (FOD). Usually the FOD is kept as long as possible relative to the FFD to reduce the amount of magnification to a minimum.

Armstrong. *Lecture Notes on the Physics of Radiology*, 1st Edn. Clinical Press Ltd.

**A 14. A.** false **B.** false **C.** true **D.** true **E.** false

All forms of EMR travel with the same velocity as light when in a vacuum. The velocity is NOT significantly less in air.
All forms of EMR obey the inverse square law only when in vacuum.
Intensity = watts per square millimetre.
The energy of X- and gamma rays = MeV. Visible light = eV.

Farr, Allisy-Roberts. *Physics for Medical Imaging*, 1st Edn. W. B. Saunders Co. Ltd.

**A 15. A.** false **B.** false **C.** true **D.** true **E.** true

In a compound filter the material with the higher atomic number should face the X-ray tube.
A compound filter normally consists of aluminium and copper.
Filters however increase the exit dose to entry dose ratio.
Filtration does not affect the maximum photon energy. The area of the X-ray spectrum and the total output of X-rays is reduced by filtration.

Farr, Allisy-Roberts. *Physics for Medical Imaging*, 1st Edn. W. B. Saunders Co. Ltd.

**A 16. A.** false **B.** true **C.** false **D.** true **E.** false

It is known as the anode heel effect.
For a given film size, the heel effect is reduced when the FFD is increased.
Placing the thicker part of the body towards the cathode side decreases the anode heel effect.

The intensity of an X-ray beam is non-uniform for 2 reasons:
i) The anode heel effect
ii) The inverse square law: X-rays at the edge of the field have further to travel.

Farr, Allisy-Roberts. *Physics for Medical Imaging*, 1st Edn. W. B. Saunders Co. Ltd.

**A** 17. **A.** true  **B.** false  **C.** false  **D.** true  **E.** false

Optical density = Log to base 10 (incident light:transmitted light).
A log scale is used as the eye responds logarithmically to the brightness of light.
Optical densities are additive, therefore, the total optical density = 2.4.

Farr, Allisy-Roberts. *Physics for Medical Imaging*, 1st Edn. W. B. Saunders Co. Ltd.

**A** 18. **A.** true  **B.** true  **C.** false  **D.** true  **E.** true

Screen unsharpness is not magnified although the image is.

Farr, Allisy-Roberts. *Physics for Medical Imaging*, 1st Edn. W. B. Saunders Co. Ltd.

**A** 19. **A.** false  **B.** false  **C.** true  **D.** true  **E.** true

Noise is reduced by increasing the number of photons absorbed in each voxel.
Noise is decreased by either increasing slice thickness or increasing the pixel size.
Increasing mA or increasing the scan time reduces noise at the expense of increased patient dose.
Noise becomes more noticeable with narrow windowing as each grey scale covers a smaller range of CT numbers, and hence there are fewer X-ray photons absorbed in each voxel.
As the available information is spread more thinly over the pixel matrix with zoom enlargement.

Farr, Allisy-Roberts. *Physics for Medical Imaging*, 1st Edn. W. B. Saunders Co. Ltd.

**A 20.** **A.** false  **B.** true  **C.** false  **D.** false  **E.** true

Only those persons whose presence is essential should remain in an X-ray room when radiation is being generated; they should stand well away from the radiation beam and preferably behind a protective screen.
For young persons and persons of reproductive capacity, gonad shields should be used in examinations which are likely to give high gonad dose, unless these shields interfere with the proposed examination.
A posteroanterior, rather than anteroposterior, projection can greatly reduce the dose to the breast.

AC2/2, AC2/10 and Regulation 12: *IRR 88*.

**A 21.** **A.** false  **B.** true  **C.** false  **D.** false  **E.** true

4 Sv to the testes causes sterility.
For stochastic effects, the probability of an effect occurring increases with dose.
A threshold of about 5 Sv produces cataracts.

Farr, Allisy-Roberts. *Physics for Medical Imaging*, 1st Edn. W. B. Saunders Co. Ltd.

**A 22.** **A.** false  **B.** true  **C.** true  **D.** false  **E.** true

Film badges are exposed without screens.
The film badge contains a thick plastic, aluminium and tin-lead filter.
Spots of intense blackening suggests exposure to a radioactive spill.

Farr, Allisy-Roberts. *Physics for Medical Imaging*, 1st Edn. W. B. Saunders Co. Ltd.

**A 23.** **A.** false  **B.** false  **C.** true  **D.** false  **E.** true

Body aprons with a protective equivalent of not less than 0.25 mm lead for X-rays up to 100 kV and not less than 0.3 mm lead for X-rays over 100 kV should be available.
Gloves and aprons should be examined thoroughly at least once a year to ensure that no cracks have developed.

An operator should be at the control panel of a CT scanner while high voltage is applied to the X-ray tube, since the equipment will not normally have an exposure switch which has to be pressed continuously.

Gloves should be available with not less than 0.25 mm lead for X-rays up to 150 kV.

Regulation 6: *IRR 88*.

**A** 24. **A.** false   **B.** false   **C.** false   **D.** true   **E.** false

Annual background radiation = 2.5 mSv.

Natural radiation contributes 85%.

Radon gas is the largest contributor to natural background radiation. This permeates through the ground into buildings.

Food and drink contribute 12%.

Farr, Allisy-Roberts. *Physics for Medical Imaging*, 1st Edn. W. B. Saunders Co. Ltd.

**A** 25. **A.** true   **B.** false   **C.** true   **D.** false   **E.** true

The GM is able to detect any ionising radiation but not able to distinguish between them.

The efficiency of detection of gamma rays is only 1%. This can be increased to 5% by the use of a lead cylinder as a cathode.

Farr, Allisy-Roberts. *Physics for Medical Imaging*, 1st Edn. W. B. Saunders Co. Ltd.

## GAMMA IMAGING

**Q 1.  Regarding gamma imaging**

A.  A multi-hole collimator consists of a lead disc, typically 25 cm thick and 400 mm in diameter

B.  A single large phosphor crystal of NaI (activated with thallium) is positioned adjacent to the collimator

C.  The gamma crystal is hygroscopic

D.  The gamma crystal absorbs about 90% of Tc-99 m gamma rays

E.  Tc-99 m emits a 190 keV gamma ray

## GAMMA IMAGING

**Q 2.  Tc-99 m is labelled to the following compounds for the following uses**

A.  Sestamibi: cardiac perfusion imaging

B.  Diphosphonates: bone imaging

C.  Hexamethyl Propylene Amine Oxime (HMPAO): imaging the liver, spleen and red bone marrow

D.  Aminodiacetic acid (HIDA): renal imaging

E.  Human serum albumin macroaggregates: imaging of the liver, spleen and red bone marrow

## FILMS AND SCREENS

**Q 3.  Regarding film storage**

A.  Film fog increases when the film is stored at low humidity

B.  Films should ideally be stored horizontally with film packets stacked on top of each other

C.  Bending the film is not detrimental to the final image quality

D.  The maximum storage temperature should be 21 degrees centigrade

E.  Films should be handled at its edges

# X-RAY INTERACTIONS

**Q 4.** **Regarding scattered radiation**

    **A.** Scattered radiation adds to the final image quality achieved

    **B.** Scatter makes up about 15% of the total number of photons emerging from a patient

    **C.** Apart from scattered radiation, the only other secondary radiation reaching the film is characteristic radiation arising from contrast media such as barium

    **D.** Increasing scatter is produced with large fields of view

    **E.** Increasing scatter is produced when irradiating thick body parts

# X-RAY TUBES

**Q 5.** **The following are true regarding the stationary anode tube**

    **A.** The 'real' focus is the area bombarded by electrons emitted from the filament

    **B.** The principal heat path is via conduction

    **C.** X-ray output is limited primarily because the anode is made of copper

    **D.** It has very limited use in diagnostic radiology

    **E.** The 'quality' of the X-ray beam will be identical to that of a rotating anode tube if both have target materials of tungsten and operate at the same kVp

# IMAGE QUALITY

**Q 6.** **The following are criteria for attaining a radiograph of satisfactory quality**

    **A.** The choice of contrast is unimportant

    **B.** A wide contrast scale should be used

    **C.** A narrow contrast scale should be used

    **D.** The contrast scale used should be such that differences between densities can be readily made

    **E.** Contrast is controlled by the choice of target material used

# X-RAY INTERACTIONS

**Q 7.** **The following statements are true**

    **A.** A material is relatively transparent to its own characteristic radiation

    **B.** Barium and iodine are suitable contrast agents as their 'K-edges' are closely related to the mean energy of the incident X-ray beam

    **C.** The total linear attenuation coefficient (LAC) is the sum of the LACs of the contributions from elastic, photoelectric and Compton scattering

    **D.** In the diagnostic imaging range, the Compton effect predominates for air, water and soft tissue

    **E.** The SI units for mass attenuation coefficient are square centimetres per gram

# FILMS AND SCREENS

**Q 8.** **The following are true**

    **A.** The speed of a film is the reciprocal of the exposure needed to produce an optical density of 1 above base + fog

    **B.** Inherent fog has typically an optical density; $D = 0.12$

    **C.** Storage conditions affect inherent fog

    **D.** Emulsions with rounded crystals are faster than those with flat crystals

    **E.** The speed of a film decreases with increasing average grain size

# IMAGE QUALITY

**Q 9.** **Regarding image quality**

    **A.** Spatial resolution (SR) of an imaging system is defined as the spatial frequency of the finest pattern in a test tool that can be resolved

    **B.** Spatial frequency is usually denoted as the number of line pairs per millimetre (lp/mm) detectable

    **C.** The SR of an X-ray film is about 100 lp/mm

    **D.** A detailed intensifying screen has an SR of about 30 lp/mm

    **E.** A fast screen has an SR of about 15 lp/mm

**Q** **10. Regarding CT artefacts**

   **A.** Cardiac motion produces streak artefacts
   **B.** In fourth-generation scanners, detector malfunction is manifest as ring artefacts
   **C.** Dental amalgam gives rise to star artefacts
   **D.** 'Cupping' occurs as a consequence of beam hardening
   **E.** Aliasing may occur at sharp and high-contrast boundaries

## RADIOACTIVITY

**Q** **11. Regarding radioactive decay**

   **A.** In beta minus decay there is no change in the atomic number, but the mass number increases by one
   **B.** In isomeric transition, the parent nucleus decays directly to the daughter nucleus by the emission of a negative beta particle
   **C.** In beta plus decay, there is no change in the atomic number, but the mass number decreases by one
   **D.** In positron emission, two photons of annihilation radiation are emitted at right angles to each other
   **E.** The SI units of radioactive decay is the becquerel (Bq), where one Bq = the number of disintegrations per minute

## GAMMA IMAGING

**Q** **12. Regarding gamma imaging**

   **A.** There are usually between 37 and 90 photomultiplier tubes (PMT) connected to the gamma crystal
   **B.** Each PMT consists of a glass envelope containing xenon gas at 4 atmospheres
   **C.** Photoelectrons emitted in a PMT undergo amplification by interacting with a series of dynodes
   **D.** The purpose of the pulse arithmetic circuit is to combine the pulses from all the PMTs and generate three separate voltage pulses
   **E.** The purpose of the pulse height analyser is to reject pulses which are either lower or higher than pre-set levels

# GAMMA IMAGING

**Q 13. Radionuclides and administered activities**

    **A.** Kr-81 m gas in lung ventilation studies: 6,000 MBq
    **B.** Tc-99 m MAG3 in renal imaging: 100 MBq
    **C.** Tc-99 m phosphonates in bone imaging: 100 MBq
    **D.** Tc-99 m DTPA in renal imaging: 80 MBq
    **E.** Tc-99 m DTPA aerosol in lung ventilation studies: 80 MBq

# X-RAY TUBES

**Q 14. Regarding quality assurance as assessed by a physicist**

    **A.** Focal spot measurement should be assessed annually
    **B.** Focal spot size is usually assessed by the pinhole method
    **C.** Beam alignment is usually assessed every 3 months
    **D.** The tolerance limits for beam alignment are +/− 2%
    **E.** X-ray tube output and kV should be assessed every 3 months

# X-RAY INTERACTIONS AND FILTERS

**Q 15. The following are true regarding the half-value thickness**

    **A.** It is the absorber thickness required to reduce the intensity of the original beam by half
    **B.** In the diagnostic energy range, the half-value thickness is usually measured in millimeters of aluminium
    **C.** Is inversely proportional to the linear attenuation coefficient
    **D.** Is a measure of the penetrating power of a beam
    **E.** The product of half-value layer and the linear attenuation coefficient is always a constant

# DOSIMETRY

**Q 16. Regarding film badge dosimetry**

    **A.** Double-emulsion film is used, one with a high gamma and one with a low gamma
    **B.** The cadmium-lead filter is used to detect exposure to neutrons
    **C.** The use of plastic, tin and aluminium filters in the film badge, allows differentiation between the penetrating radiations used in both radiotherapy and in the range of energies usual in radiodiagnosis

Exam 5

Questions

**D.** Latent imaging fading does not occur if there is a delay between exposure and development of a film badge

**E.** Control films must be processed with each batch of film dosimeters going through the processor

## FILMS AND SCREENS

### Q 17. Regarding modulation transfer function (MTF)

**A.** Has units of line pairs per millimeter

**B.** Is normally greater than one

**C.** MTF is a ratio of the information recorded to the information available

**D.** The MTF can be used to compare the resolving power of one imaging system versus another

**E.** A 10% response on an MTF curve is the definition of the resolving power of an imaging system

## DOSIMETRY

### Q 18. Concerning thermoluminescent materials in dosimetry (TLD)

**A.** The electron traps in the forbidden zone of thermoluminescent materials are normally full

**B.** The electron traps are well below the conduction band

**C.** Electrons in the electron traps enter the conduction band when the material is heated to 100 degrees centigrade

**D.** When the TLD material is heated, the total amount of light emitted is proportional to the amount of radiation absorbed

**E.** The material most commonly used in TLDs is zinc cadmium sulphide

## X-RAY INTERACTIONS

### Q 19. The linear attenuation coefficient of an X-ray beam

**A.** Is defined as the reduction in intensity per unit area of absorber

**B.** Is greater in bone than in fat at 35 keV

**C.** Can be used to calculate half-value thickness (HVT)

**D.** Applies to both mono- and polychromatic radiations

**E.** Is a constant for a monochromatic beam

# RADIATION PROTECTION

**Q 20.** **The National Radiation Protection Board (NRPB) recommends that the following views should not be part of a 'routine' X-ray examination**

A. Lateral chest view
B. Coned view of the pituitary fossa
C. Oblique views of the cervical spine
D. Post-micturition film of an IVU
E. A post-evacuation film after a barium enema

# RADIATION PROTECTION

**Q 21.** **Radiation Protection**

A. The relative biological effectiveness (RBE) of radiation is the ratio of the number of Grays of two radiation qualities that give the same biological effect on the same material in the same time
B. The RBE for X-rays is 10
C. The annual effective dose limit for a radiation worker (18 and over) is ten times greater than that for a member of the public
D. Natural background radiation contributes 5 mSv to the annual whole-body dose per person in the UK
E. The largest contributor to natural background radiation is radon and thoron

# RADIATION PROTECTION

**Q 22.** **Regarding dose limits**

A. The annual effective dose limit for members of staff, 18 years of age and older, is 20 mSv
B. The annual effective dose limit for members of the public or visitors is 15 mSv
C. The annual equivalent dose limit to the eyes for a trainee aged less than 18 years is 50 mSv
D. The annual dose limit to the extremity for a member of staff, 18 years of age and older, is 500 mSv
E. Staff are designated as classified if they exceed 20% of any annual dose limit

## RADIATION PROTECTION

**Q 23. Ionising Radiation (IRMER) Regulations 2000**

A. All persons directing an exposure need to be adequately trained in radiation protection matters
B. IRMER does not apply to scientific research for in vitro studies
C. The responsibility for an exposure lies with the person clinically directing it
D. The ALARA principle does not apply in IRMER
E. No exposure should be directed unless its introduction produces a positive net benefit

## RADIATION PROTECTION

**Q 24. The following UK legislation is appropriate for the individuals described**

A. Staff and members of the public: Ionising Radiation Regulations 1999 (IRR 99)
B. Patients: IR(ME)R 2000
C. Staff and members of the public: Radioactive Substances Act 1993
D. Patients: The Medicines (Administration of Radioactive Substances) Regulations 1978: M(ARS)R 78
E. Approved Codes of Practice and Guidance Notes; these do not play a part in UK legislation

## RADIATION PROTECTION

**Q 25. Radiation protection**

A. In the UK the average annual total effective dose (ED) to the population is 2.5 Sv
B. 5% of the average annual total ED is from medical investigations or treatment
C. Medical staff in a radiology department commonly receive an annual total ED twice that of the national average
D. Potassium-40 is a major contributor to the ED from background radiation arising through the ground
E. The residents of Cornwall receive an annual total ED seven times the national average

**A 1.**   **A.** false   **B.** true   **C.** true   **D.** true   **E.** false

Multi-hole collimator: the lead disc is typically 25 mm thick,
and is drilled with about 20,000 hexagonal or circular
holes.
As the crystal is hygroscopic, it is encapsulated in an aluminium
cylinder to protect it from changes in temperature, light and
atmosphere.
Tc-99 m emits a 140 keV gamma ray.

Farr, Allisy-Roberts. *Physics for Medical Imaging*, 1st Edn. W. B. Saunders
Co. Ltd.

**A 2.**   **A.** true   **B.** true   **C.** false   **D.** false   **E.** false

HMPAO: cerebral imaging.
HIDA: biliary imaging.
Macroaggregates of albumin: lung perfusion imaging.

Farr, Allisy-Roberts. *Physics for Medical Imaging*, 1st Edn. W. B. Saunders Co.
Ltd.

**A 3.**   **A.** false   **B.** false   **C.** false   **D.** true   **E.** true

When film is stored it should be stored at low humidity, side on
and care must be taken not to flex the film. Increased humidity
tends to increase film fog.

Curry, Thomas. *Christensen's Physics of Diagnostic Radiology*, 4th Edn.
Williams & Wilkins (Europe) Ltd.

**A 4.**   **A.** false   **B.** false   **C.** true   **D.** true   **E.** true

Scattered radiation serves no useful value, and if it reaches
the film impairs film quality. It decreases contrast
resolution.

Scatter makes up about 50–90% of the total number of photons emerging from a patient.

Armstrong. *Lecture Notes on the Physics of Radiology*, 1st Edn. Clinical Press Ltd., 1990.

**A 5.** **A.** true **B.** true **C.** false **D.** true **E.** true

The X-ray output is limited from stationary anode tubes due to the heat limitation from tube-loading characteristics.

Curry, Thomas. *Christensen's Physics of Diagnostic Radiology*, 4th Edn. Williams & Wilkins (Europe) Ltd.

**A 6.** **A.** false **B.** false **C.** false **D.** true **E.** false

Naturally the use of contrast media is important, hence its extensive use in radiology.
Radiographic contrast is dependent on many factors such as selection of kV, mA, patient factors and film factors.

Curry, Thomas. *Christensen's Physics of Diagnostic Radiology*, 4th Edn. Williams & Wilkins (Europe) Ltd.

**A 7.** **A.** true **B.** true **C.** true **D.** true **E.** true

Farr, Allisy-Roberts. *Physics for Medical Imaging*, 1st Edn. W. B. Saunders Co. Ltd.

**A 8.** **A.** true **B.** true **C.** false **D.** false **E.** false

Inherent fog arises from some silver halide crystals acquiring latent images during manufacture, and also from the film base absorbing light when viewed. Storage conditions affect additional fog.
Emulsion film with flat crystals are faster than those with rounded crystals.
Film speed increases with increasing average grain size.

Farr, Allisy-Roberts. *Physics for Medical Imaging*, 1st Edn. W. B. Saunders Co. Ltd.

**A 9.** **A.** true **B.** true **C.** true **D.** false **E.** false

Detail screen: SR – 10 lp/mm.
Fast screen: SR – 5 lp/mm.

Farr, Allisy-Roberts. *Physics for Medical Imaging*, 1st Edn. W. B. Saunders Co. Ltd.

**A 10.** **A.** true **B.** true **C.** true **D.** true **E.** true

Ring artefacts usually signify detector malfunction in third-generation scanners.
Star artefacts may also occur with metal implants or high-density contrast medium.

Farr. Allisy-Roberts. *Physics for Medical Imaging*, 1st Edn. W. B. Saunders Co. Ltd.

**A 11.** **A.** false **B.** false **C.** false **D.** false **E.** false

Beta minus: there is no change in mass number, the atomic number increases by one.
Isomeric transition: the daughter nucleus remains in a metastable state for a variable length of time, prior to emitting a gamma ray and decaying to the ground state.
Beta plus: there is no change in mass number, the atomic number decreases by one.
The photons of annihilation radiation are emitted in opposite directions.
1 Bq = 1 disintegration per second.

Farr, Allisy-Roberts. *Physics for Medical Imaging*, W. B. Saunders Co. Ltd.

**A 12.** **A.** true **B.** false **C.** true **D.** true **E.** true

Each PMT consists of an evacuated glass envelope.
Typically a single photoelectron may be amplified by a factor of 1 million.
Three voltage pulses are generated: X, Y and Z. X and Y give positional information. The Z pulse is proportional to the gamma ray energy absorbed.
The pulse height analyser may be set to only let through those pulses which lie within a window of $+/-10\%$ of the photopeak energy.

**A** **13.** **A.** true **B.** true **C.** false **D.** true **E.** true

Tc-99 m phosphonates: administered activity 600 MBq.

**A** **14.** **A.** true **B.** false **C.** false **D.** true **E.** true

The pinhole method is the oldest method for assessing focal spot size, and is now outdated. It could only be used for focal spots greater than 0.3 mm. Focal spot size is now assessed via a 'STAR' test tool.
Beam alignment is assessed annually.

**A** **15.** **A.** true **B.** true **C.** true **D.** true **E.** true

HVL $\times$ linear attenuation coefficient = 0.693

**A** **16.** **A.** true **B.** true **C.** true **D.** false **E.** true

The slow emulsion allows extension of the range of measurement up to 100 Sv in case of large accidental exposures. The different filters allow a distinction to be made as to whether the exposure resulted from beta emission, high or low-energy X-rays or gamma emission.
Latent image fading can occur, particularly in humid conditions, if there is a delay between exposure and development. This is due to the gradual loss of electrons which formed the latent image by conversion of the sensitivity speck to metallic silver. The processing conditions have a critical affect on film badges and so control films must be processed with each batch of film dose meters.

**A** 17. **A.** false **B.** false **C.** true **D.** true **E.** true

Modulation transfer function has no units.
As the recorded information can never exceed the available information, the MTF is always less than one.

Curry, Thomas. Christensen's Physics of Diagnostic Radiology, 4th Edn. Williams & Wilkins (Europe) Ltd.

**A** 18. **A.** false **B.** true **C.** false **D.** true **E.** false

Thermoluminescent materials contain electron traps which are normally empty.
Electron traps are well below the conduction band, so there is little chance at ordinary temperatures of electrons being elevated into the conduction band.
Electrons enter the conduction band when the material is heated to 200–300 °C.
The material most commonly used in TLDs is lithium fluoride powder.

Armstrong. *Lecture Notes on the Physics of Radiology*, 1st Edn. Clinical Press Ltd., 1990.

**A** 19. **A.** false **B.** true **C.** true **D.** false **E.** true

The linear attenuation coefficient is defined as the fractional reduction in intensity per unit length of absorber. The units are per centimetre.
The HVT equals 0.693 divided by linear attenuation coefficient.
Linear attenuation coefficient applies to monochromatic radiation only, and is specific both for the energy of the X-ray beam and for the type of absorber.

Armstrong. *Lecture Notes on the Physics of Radiology*, 1st Edn. Clinical Press Ltd., 1990.

**A** 20. **A.** true **B.** true **C.** true **D.** true **E.** true

The NRPB also recommends that the following views should not be performed as part of 'routine' radiography:
1) Flexion and extension views of the cervical spine
2) Coned L5/S1 and obliques of the lumbar spine
3) Skyline and tunnel views of the knees

4) 1-min film from an IVU.

The NRPB also recommends the following:
i) The occipito-mental view should be the only view performed when examining the sinuses.
ii) The submento-vertical view should not be routinely performed when examining the skull.
iii) An AP odontoid peg view should not be taken unless there is a history of trauma.

Report by the Royal College of Radiologists and the National Radiation Protection Board (1990). *Patient Dose Reduction in Diagnostic Radiology.* National Radiation Protection Board.

**A** **21.** **A.** true **B.** false **C.** false **D.** false **E.** true

The RBE for X-rays is 1.
The annual effective dose limit for a radiation worker (18 and over) is 20 mSv; that for a member of the public is 1 mSv.
The average annual whole-body dose per person in the UK due to natural background radiation is approximately 2.5 mSv.

Curry, Thomas. *Christensen's Physics of Diagnostic Radiology,* 4th Edn. Williams & Wilkins (Europe) Ltd.

**A** **22.** **A.** false **B.** false **C.** true **D.** true **E.** false

Annual dose limit for members of the public = 1 mSv.
Exceeding 30% of any annual dose limit results in the individual being 'classified'.

Farr, Allisy-Roberts. *Physics for Medical Imaging,* 1st Edn. W. B. Saunders Co. Ltd.

**A** **23.** **A.** true **B.** true **C.** true **D.** false **E.** true

The ALARA principle should always be applied when directing ionising radiation.

*The Ionising Radiation (Medical Exposure) Regulations 2000*

**A** **24.** **A.** true **B.** true **C.** true **D.** true **E.** false

The Approved Codes of Practice and Guidance give detailed and practical recommendations on how the legislation should be implemented locally in X-ray and nuclear medicine departments.

Farr, Allisy-Roberts. *Physics for Medical Imaging,* 1st Edn. W. B. Saunders Co. Ltd.

A 25. **A.** false   **B.** false   **C.** false   **D.** false   **E.** false

The average annual total ED to the population is 2.5 mSv.
Medical investigations contribute about 14% of the average annual ED.
Medical staff, through adequate shielding, should receive very low doses, almost on par with the general population.
Potassium-40 is a natural radionuclide in food. The major contributors from the ground are radon and thoron.
People in Cornwall receive an annual total ED about three times the national average.

Curry, Thomas. *Christensen's Physics of Diagnostic Radiology*, 4th Edn. Williams & Wilkins (Europe) Ltd.

## X-RAY TUBES

**Q 1.  The line focus principle**

A.  Maximises the area over which heat is generated
B.  Minimises the geometric unsharpness of an image
C.  Ensures that the effective focal spot is larger than the true focal spot
D.  Ensures that the real focal spot is larger than the effective focal spot
E.  In the majority of X-ray tubes, the target is at an angle within the range of 6–20 degrees

## DOSIMETRY

**Q 2.  The following are true**

A.  The absorbed dose is the energy deposited per unit area of a material
B.  Kerma is the kinetic energy released per unit mass of an irradiated material
C.  A 'thimble' chamber can be used to measure air kerma
D.  A standard free air chamber is commonly used in most departments to measure air kerma
E.  Silver bromide is used for dosimetry in thermoluminescent dosimeters (TLD)

## TOMOGRAPHY

**Q 3.  Regarding tomography**

A.  The greater the tomographic angle of swing, the thinner the cut
B.  Only structures at right angles to the film are imaged sharply
C.  The further a structure is from the pivot plane, the greater the movement blur

D. Tomography is most useful when imaging structures of high inherent contrast
  E. Larger tomographic angles are used in zonography as compared to tomography

# FILMS AND SCREENS

**Q 4. The following statements are true**

  A. Increasing developer temperature increases speed of development and reduces fog
  B. Increasing the developer temperature may cause an initial increase in film gamma
  C. Developer concentration and developing time have little effect on the quality of film development
  D. Quality assurance (QA) of a processing unit may be carried out with a sensitometer
  E. In QA of a processing unit, a daily variation in densities of 30% is acceptable

# ANGIOGRAPHY

**Q 5. Digital subtraction angiography (DSA)**

  A. The mask image is taken before the administration of contrast
  B. A small field image intensifier with good contrast resolution is required
  C. Following subtraction the signal to noise ratio (SNR)is reduced
  D. In energy subtraction, a mask image is routinely taken
  E. In hybrid subtraction, two energy subtracted pre-contrast images and two energy subtracted post-contrast images are temporally subtracted from each other

# CT

**Q 6. Regarding spiral helical scanning**

  A. Partial volume artefacts are reduced compared to conventional axial scanning
  B. Slice to slice misregistration is exaggerated compared to conventional axial scanning

**C.** 'Pitch' is the slice thickness (mm) divided by the distance (mm) moved by the table during one rotation of the tube

**D.** When a pitch of greater than 2:1 is used, artefacts may arise due to gaps in the volume data acquisition

**E.** Heat loading of the tube is greater with conventional axial scanning compared to helical scanning

## GAMMA IMAGING

**Q 7.** **Regarding collimators used in gamma imaging**

**A.** The greater the number of holes in a collimator, the better the spatial resolution (SR)

**B.** The wider the holes in a collimator – improved SR

**C.** The shorter the holes in a collimator – improved SR

**D.** Spatial resolution and sensitivity of a collimator are inversely related

**E.** The SR of a collimator is improved if it is placed as close as possible to the patient

## GAMMA IMAGING

**Q 8.** **Regarding positron emission tomography (PET)**

**A.** The process of annihilation radiation produces two photons of 511 keV moving in opposite directions

**B.** The detectors usually used are NaI (activated with traces of thallium)

**C.** The photomultiplier tubes are coupled to a parallel hole collimator

**D.** The effective dose to the patient is much higher than in planar gamma imaging

**E.** The spatial resolution in PET may be 5 mm or less

## MAMMOGRAPHY

**Q 9.** **Regarding quality assurance performed by a radiographer in mammography**

**A.** Processor performance and sensitometry should be assessed daily

**B.** Automatic exposure control should be assessed weekly

C. X-ray kV accuracy and output should be assessed weekly
D. Screen film contact should be assessed monthly
E. A full change of chemicals and servicing of processor is suggested every 4 weeks for a screening programme

# RADIOACTIVITY

**Q 10. Regarding radioactivity**

A. The unit of radioactivity is the becquerel (Bq), where 1 Bq is 1 disintegration per second
B. The concentration of radioactivity is measured in Bq/kg
C. At a temperature of absolute zero the radioactive decay process is unaffected
D. In stable heavy nuclei, there are an excess number of neutrons relative to the number of protons
E. X-rays have a greater maximum possible energy than gamma rays

# X-RAY INTERACTIONS AND FILTERS

**Q 11. Regarding the filtration of X-rays**

A. Tissue contrast is increased
B. The photoelectric effect predominates
C. A beryllium window results in less attenuation of the beam compared to a glass window
D. When aluminium is being used as a filter facing an anode, a backing filter is also required
E. For undercouch fluoroscopy, 2.5–4 mm of aluminium is the recommended added tube filtration

# DOSIMETRY

**Q 12. Dosimetry**

A. A thimble chamber has an atomic number (Z) approximately equal to that of air
B. An exposure rate meter requires a resistor in parallel to a voltmeter
C. In an exposure meter, the outer wall of an ionisation chamber is connected to the capacitor

D. The response of an ionisation chamber increases with increasing wall thickness

E. The use of a lead cylinder cathode in a Geiger-Muller tube, increases the detection of efficiency of gamma rays

## FILMS AND SCREENS

Q 13. **Concerning X-ray film**

A. The supercoat consists of a thin later of polyester

B. Film speed is a reciprocal of the exposure needed to produce a density of 1 above base plus fog

C. Exposing a film to bright light after fixation will destroy the image of the film

D. Fog is more noticeable at low densities

E. Incomplete washing of the film following fixation will result in the film developing a brown layer of silver sulphide

## X-RAY TUBES

Q 14. **In a rotating anode tube, the X-ray tube assembly is primarily immersed in oil for the following reasons**

A. To provide lubrication for the rotating anode

B. To filter the X-ray beam

C. To assist in the cooling of the anode following an exposure

D. To provide electrical insulation

E. To provide mechanical protection to the X-ray tube assembly

## FILMS AND SCREENS

Q 15. **The following are true**

A. The gamma of a film refers to the maximum slope of the shoulder region of the characteristic curve

B. High gamma films have a narrow exposure latitude

C. Low gamma films have a narrow exposure latitude

D. Low gamma films have low inherent film contrast

E. The optical density of a film plotted against the reciprocal of the exposure given to that film is known as the characteristic curve

# IMAGE QUALITY

**Q 16. Regarding film processing**

   **A.** Films are washed with water prior to fixing

   **B.** The developer is kept alkaline to keep the pH between 9.6 and 10.6

   **C.** Glutaraldehyde in the developer acts as an anti-fogging agent

   **D.** The purpose of the fixer is to immediately stop any further development of latent image centres

   **E.** The fixer contains aluminium salts which harden the film and reduce drying time

# FLUOROSCOPY

**Q 17. Regarding the resolution of an image intensifier**

   **A.** The centre of the image intensifier screen has a brighter image than the periphery

   **B.** The periphery of an image intensifier screen has a better resolution than the central field

   **C.** There is less geometric distortion at the periphery of the intensifier screen compared to the centre

   **D.** The effects of geometric distortion are more pronounced in small field intensifiers

   **E.** Electrons at the periphery of the intensifier field are less accurately focused than those at the centre and produce unequal magnification

# X-RAY INTERACTIONS

**Q 18. Regarding the interaction of X-rays or gamma rays with tissue**

   **A.** Produce secondary electrons

   **B.** Are more for higher atomic number materials

   **C.** At lower energies, the interaction occurs in a manner which is predominantly inversely proportional to the square of their energy

   **D.** Scatter predominantly in a forward direction

   **E.** The interaction may occur with either free or bound electrons

# X-RAY TUBES

## Q 19. In diagnostic radiology

A. Dental tubes usually have rotating anodes
B. Fine and coarse focus are selected by the application of a different current to a single filament
C. In linear tomography the greater the angle of swing the thicker the cut
D. When multiple simultaneous tomographic cuts are made, all the film screen combinations have the same sensitivity
E. Rotating anode tubes do not need to be filled with oil

# RADIATION PROTECTION

## Q 20. The following are non-stochastic effects

A. Cataract formation
B. Skin erythema
C. Sterility
D. Leukaemia
E. Muscular dystrophy

# RADIATION PROTECTION

## Q 21. The following statements are true

A. In fluoroscopy with an undercouch tube, drapes of at least 0.35 mm lead equivalence are attached to the lower edge
B. In gamma imaging, body aprons should have at least 0.5 mm lead equivalence
C. 2.5 mm lead equivalence is often satisfactory for use in the walls, doors and windows of an X-ray room
D. 60 mm of concrete is approximately equal to 1 mm lead equivalence
E. 12 mm of barium plaster is approximately equal to 1 mm lead equivalence

# RADIATION PROTECTION

## Q 22. The following statements are true

A. In an X-ray tube, the total filtration should never be less than the equivalent of 0.5 mm aluminium
B. For radiography of the chest, the focal spot to skin distance should not be less than 30 cm

C. In hypocycloidal tomography and cerebral angiography, the use of lead or lead-containing shields should be considered for protection of the lens of the patient's eye
D. During fluoroscopy, palpation with the hand should only be undertaken with an overcouch tube
E. A protective glove with a lead equivalent thickness of at least 0.25 mm should be used for X-rays up to 150 kV

# RADIATION PROTECTION

**Q 23. Regarding tissue weighting factors (Wt)**

A. Gonads: Wt 0.2
B. Red bone marrow: Wt 0.12
C. Breast: Wt 0.12
D. Lung: Wt 0.05
E. Thyroid: Wt 0.05

# RADIATION PROTECTION

**Q 24. Regarding dosimetry**

A. Lithium fluoride (LiF) may be used as the phosphor material in a thermoluminescent dosimeter (TLD)
B. TLDs are suitable for finger dosimetry
C. When using film badges it is not possible to identify the type and energy of an exposure
D. LiF chips are annealed in order to remove any residual stored energy from a previous exposure
E. TLDs are not affective over a wide range of exposure doses

# RADIATION PROTECTION

**Q 25. The following statements are true**

A. The inherent filtration of every tube assembly should be marked permanently and clearly on the tube housing
B. For normal diagnostic work, the total filtration of the beam should be equivalent to not less than 2.5 mm of aluminium of which 1.5 mm should be permanent
C. All radiographic X-ray equipment should be provided with properly aligned adjustable beam-limiting devices to keep

the radiation beam within the limits of the X-ray film selected for each examination

**D.** The housing and supporting plates of an X-ray image intensifier should provide shielding equivalent of least 1 mm lead for 100 kV

**E.** In mammography, the total permanent filtration should never be less than 0.3 mm molybdenum

**A 1.**   **A.** true   **B.** true   **C.** false   **D.** true   **E.** true

Curry, Thomas. *Christensen's Physics of Diagnostic Radiology*, 4th Edn. Williams & Wilkins (Europe) Ltd.

**A 2.**   **A.** false   **B.** true   **C.** true   **D.** false   **E.** false

Absorbed dose is the energy deposited per unit mass (J/kg). Kerma and absorbed dose are more or less synonymous with each other and are measured in Grays (1 Gy = 1 J/kg). Standard free air chambers are 800 times larger than thimble chambers and are therefore impracticable for use in most departments. Silver bromide is used in film badge dosimetry.

Farr, Allisy-Roberts. *Physics for Medical Imaging*, 1st Edn. W. B. Saunders Co. Ltd.

**A 3.**   **A.** true   **B.** false   **C.** true   **D.** true   **E.** false

Structures parallel to the film are imaged sharply, those at right angles tend to be blurred to a greater extent. Tomography is useful when imaging, for example, the inner ear and in pyelography. Zonography: 5–10 degrees, tomography: 30–50 degrees.

Farr, Allisy-Roberts. *Physics for Medical Imaging*, 1st Edn. W. B. Saunders Co. Ltd.

**A 4.**   **A.** false   **B.** true   **C.** false   **D.** true   **E.** false

Speed of development is increased by increasing the developer temperature but there is also an associated increase in fog. When the developer temperature rises above a temperature recommended by the manufacturer, there is an increase in fog which reduces the average film gamma.

Increasing developer concentration and increasing developing time have similar affects to those of increasing developer temperature.

QA involves measuring the density, following processing, of a film on which a step wedge image is pre-exposed.

In QA a 0–15% daily variation in densities are acceptable.

Farr, Allisy-Roberts. *Physics for Medical Imaging*, 1st Edn. W. B. Saunders Co. Ltd.

**A 5.**    **A.** true   **B.** false   **C.** true   **D.** false   **E.** true

A large field intensifier (300 mm) is needed.

Following subtraction, the signals subtract but the noise is reinforced, thereby reducing the SNR.

With energy subtraction, rapid switching between a high kV e.g., 140 and a lower kV e.g., 65, avoids the need for a mask image.

In hybrid subtraction, the temporal subtraction would eliminate bone, for example, leaving the vessel filled with contrast medium.

Farr, Allisy-Roberts. *Physics for Medical Imaging*, 1st Edn. W. B. Saunders Co. Ltd.

**A 6.**    **A.** true   **B.** false   **C.** false   **D.** true   **E.** false

Partial volume artefacts are reduced since the volume acquisition data can be reconstructed in small steps.

As there is volume acquisition of data, the problem of slice to slice misregistration is overcome, especally in the region of the diaphragm.

'Pitch' is defined as the distance moved by the table during one rotation divided by the slice thickness.

As there is no cooling period between slices in helical scanning, heat loading of the tube is greater than in conventional axial scanning.

Farr, Allisy-Roberts. *Physics for Medical Imaging*, 1st Edn. W. B. Saunders Co. Ltd.

**A 7.**    **A.** false   **B.** false   **C.** false   **D.** true   **E.** true

The resolution deteriorates but the sensitivity improves with increasing the number of holes in the collimator.

There is improved sensitivity at the expense of decreased SR when using collimators with both wider and shorter holes.

Farr, Allisy-Roberts. *Physics for Medical Imaging*, 1st Edn. W. B. Saunders Co. Ltd.

**A 8.** **A.** true  **B.** false  **C.** false  **D.** false  **E.** true

Bismuth germinate is usually used for the detectors.
Collimators are not routinely used in PET imaging
The effective dose to a patient is much the same as in routine gamma imaging as the short half-lives of the radionuclides used compensates for their beta emission.
The resolution in PET is better than in SPECT and is the same at all depths in a patient. In SPECT, however, spatial resolution worsens with increasing depth.

Farr, Allisy-Roberts. *Physics for Medical Imaging*, 1st Edn. W. B. Saunders Co. Ltd.

**A 9.** **A.** true  **B.** false  **C.** true  **D.** false  **E.** true

Automatic exposure control: Exposure of a 4 cm perspex phantom should yield a film giving a consistent optical density from a consistent exposure mAs. This should be checked on a daily basis.
Screen film contact should be assessed every 3 months.

Thomas. The Technique of Mammography – Quality Assurance. *Jarvis Screening Diagnostic and National Training Centre Manual.*

**A 10.** **A.** true  **B.** false  **C.** true  **D.** true  **E.** false

The concentration of radioactivity is measured in Bq/ml. Bq/kg is a measure of the specific activity of a radioactive sample.
Gamma rays have a greater maximum possible energy than X-rays. This is because gamma rays originate at a nuclear level whilst X-rays originate from changes in the electron shells.

Curry, Thomas. *Christensen's Physics of Diagnostic Radiology*, 4th Edn. Williams & Wilkins (Europe) Ltd.

**A 11.** **A.** false  **B.** true  **C.** true  **D.** false  **E.** true

As the mean kV of the beam is increased with filtration, tissue contrast is reduced.

No backing filter is required as the characteristic radiation emitted by the aluminium is of low energy (1.5 kV) and this is absorbed in air.

Curry, Thomas. *Christensen's Physics of Diagnostic Radiology*, 4th Edn. Williams & Wilkins (Europe) Ltd.

A 12. **A.** true **B.** true **C.** false **D.** false **E.** true

Z of air is 7.62 and that of the wall is 6. However, as the central electrode has a Z of about 13, the Z of the combined ionisation chamber (IC) approximates to that of air.
In an exposure meter a capacitor is used in parallel to the voltmeter and the central electrode of the chamber is connected to the capacitor.
Above a certain wall thickness, the response of the chamber decreases due to attenuation of the beam by the wall itself.
The efficiency of detection increases from about 1–5% when using a lead cylinder cathode.

Curry, Thomas. *Christensen's Physics of Diagnostic Radiology*, 4th Edn. Williams & Wilkins (Europe) Ltd.

A 13. **A.** false **B.** true **C.** false **D.** true **E.** true

The supercoat is usually made of gelatin.
The image would be destroyed if the film was exposed to light prior to fixing.

Curry, Thomas. *Christensen's Physics of Diagnostic Radiology*, 4th Edn. Williams & Wilkins Ltd.

A 14. **A.** false **B.** false **C.** false **D.** true **E.** false

Whilst the use of the oil does provide a degree of filtration and allows the transfer of heat by radiation from the anode, the principal reason that the X-ray tube assembly is immersed in oil is for the electrical insulation it provides.

Curry, Thomas. *Christensen's Physics of Diagnostic Radiology*, 4th Edn. Williams & Wilkins (Europe) Ltd.

**A.** false **B.** true **C.** false **D.** true **E.** false

The gamma of a film refers to the maximum slope of the straight-line portion of the characteristic curve. The steeper the straight-line portion, the higher the gamma and vice versa.
Low gamma film has a wide exposure latitude.
The characteristic curve is formed by plotting the optical density against the log of the exposure given to the film.

Armstrong. *Lecture Notes on the Physics of Radiology*, 1st Edn. Clinical Press Ltd., 1990.

**A** 16. **A.** false **B.** true **C.** false **D.** true **E.** true

Immediately following the developer, the film goes straight into the fixer tank after which it is washed with water to remove the silver bromide in solution and fixer chemicals. Fixer has an acid pH of 4–5.
Glutaraldehyde is a hardening agent.

Armstrong. *Lecture Notes on the Physics of Radiology*, 1st Edn. Clinical Press Ltd., 1990.

**A** 17. **A.** true **B.** false **C.** false **D.** false **E.** true

Electrons at the periphery of the intensification field are less accurately focused than those at the centre of the magnification field.
This has the following consequences: the centre of the image intensifier screen has a brighter image, better resolution and less geometric distortion. These features are worse with large field intensifiers.

Armstrong. *Lecture Notes on the Physics of Radiology*, 1st Edn. Clinical Press Ltd., 1990.

**A** 18. **A.** true **B.** true **C.** false **D.** false **E.** true

At lower energies, the photoelectric effect is predominant. Hence the interactions are approximately inversely proportional to the cube of the energy.

Exam 6

Answers

There is no bias toward forward scattering. Scattering can occur in any direction, but in general the larger the angle of deflection of a scattered photon the greater the energy lost by that photon.

Curry, Thomas. *Christensen's Physics of Diagnostic Radiology*, 4th Edn. Williams & Wilkins (Europe) Ltd.

A 19. **A.** false   **B.** false   **C.** false   **D.** false   **E.** false

Dental X-ray tubes usually use stationary anodes.
Fine and coarse focus are selected by energising two different filaments.
The greater the angle of swing of an X-ray tube, the thinner the tomographic cut.
In multiple simultaneous tomography the film screen combination are of increasing sensitivity.
The insulating oil in a rotating anode tube plays an important role in the heat pathway of the rotating anode tubes.

Curry, Thomas. *Christensen's Physics of Diagnostic Radiology*, 4th Edn. Williams & Wilkins (Europe) Ltd.

A 20. **A.** true   **B.** true   **C.** true   **D.** false   **E.** false

Leukaemia is a stochastic effect.
Muscular dystrophy is a genetically inherited condition.

Farr, Allisy-Roberts. *Physics for Medical Imaging*, 1st Edn. W. B. Saunders Co. Ltd.

A 21. **A.** false   **B.** false   **C.** true   **D.** false   **E.** true

The drapes should have at least 0.5 mm of lead equivalence.
Body aprons used in diagnostic radiology are essentially ineffective against the higher photon energies encountered in nuclear medicine.
120 mm of concrete is approximately equal to 1 mm lead equivalence.

Farr, Allisy-Roberts. *Physics for Medical Imaging*, 1st Edn. W. B. Saunders Co. Ltd.

**A.** true   **B.** false   **C.** true   **D.** false   **E.** true

The focal spot to skin distance should never be less than 30 cm, and preferably not less than 45 cm when stationary equipment is used. For radiography of the chest the distance should not be less than 60 cm.

During fluoroscopy, palpation with the hand should be reduced to the minimum. It should only be undertaken on the image receptor side of the patient and therefore should not be carried out at all with an overcouch tube.

Regulation 12 and Regulation 6: *IRR 88*.

**A** 23. **A.** true   **B.** true   **C.** false   **D.** false   **E.** true

Breast: Wt 0.05.
Lung: Wt 0.12.

Farr, Allisy-Roberts. *Physics for Medical Imaging*, 1st Edn. W. B. Saunders Co. Ltd.

**A** 24. **A.** true   **B.** true   **C.** false   **D.** true   **E.** false

With film badges, it is possible to identify the type and energy of an exposure due to the presence of the double-coated emulsion and the various filters in the badge itself.

TLDs are affective over a very wide range of doses (0.1–2,000 mSv).

Farr, Allisy-Roberts. *Physics for Medical Imaging*, 1st Edn. W. B. Saunders Co. Ltd.

**A** 25. **A.** true   **B.** true   **C.** true   **D.** false   **E.** false

The housing and supporting plates of an X-ray image intensifier should provide shielding equivalent to at least 2 mm lead for 100 kV. From 100–150 kV an additional lead equivalent of 0.01 mm/kV is required. The lead equivalence should be clearly stated on the equipment.

In mammography the total permanent filtration should never be less than 0.03 mm molybdenum (equivalent to 0.5 mm aluminium).

*AC1/185, AC2/7, AC1/184, AC2/12: IRR 88*.

## IMAGE QUALITY

**Q 1. Scatter radiation**

    **A.** Reducing the field area reduces scatter production

    **B.** Applying compression reduces scatter production

    **C.** Use of a grid increases the amount of scatter reaching the film screen combination

    **D.** Use of an air-gap technique decreases the amount of scatter reaching the film due to absorption of photons within the air gap

    **E.** Use of a lower kV produces more forward scatter

## FILMS AND SCREENS

**Q 2. Regarding intensifying screens**

    **A.** Film screen combinations are more sensitive to X-ray exposure than film alone

    **B.** The use of screens reduces patient dose

    **C.** The use of screens reduces exposure times and consequently decreases movement unsharpness

    **D.** The use of screens reduces tube loading

    **E.** The use of screens increases film gamma

## MAMMOGRAPHY

**Q 3. Mammography**

    **A.** In mammography, a molybdenum filter is used primarily to remove the characteristic radiation produced at a molybdenum anode

    **B.** A single rare earth front screen is usually used

    **C.** For macro-radiography, a focal spot size of 0.1 mm is used

    **D.** Compression of the breast only serves to cause discomfort to the patient

    **E.** Films with a gamma of about 3 are used

# FILMS AND SCREENS

**Q 4.** **Intensifying screens**

    **A.** Increase film speed

    **B.** Improve resolution when compared to film exposed directly to X-rays

    **C.** Have an increased modulation transfer function when used with magnification

    **D.** Increase film contrast

    **E.** When using green-emitting phosphors, they are associated with a greater cross-over of light compared with the use of blue-emitting phosphors

# X-RAY INTERACTIONS

**Q 5.** **Regarding the photoelectric affect**

    **A.** The entire energy of the incident photon is transferred to an orbital electron

    **B.** Following the ejection of an electron, the vacancy is filled by an outer shell electron

    **C.** It is the predominant X-ray interaction in iodinated contrast media

    **D.** It is the predominant X-ray interaction in intensifying screens

    **E.** It is the predominant mechanism by which an aluminium filter removes low-energy photons

# THE ATOM

**Q 6.** **Electromagnetic radiation**

    **A.** Includes infra-red light

    **B.** Includes radio waves

    **C.** Can behave both as a wave and as a particle

    **D.** Includes alpha emission

    **E.** Has energy that is proportional to its wavelength

# X-RAY TUBES

**Q 7.** **Tube rating**

    **A.** Is the maximum value of mA that can be achieved for any given value of kV, exposure time and focal spot size

**B.** It is the limit of power that can be put into the system

**C.** Is restricted by the amount of heat that builds up in the system

**D.** Decreases as the focal spot size increases

**E.** Is equal to $0.7 \times kV \times mA \times$ seconds for a three-phase generator

## IMAGE QUALITY

**Q 8. Image quality**

**A.** Under good viewing conditions an optical density difference of 0.04 can be seen on an X-ray film

**B.** 'True' fog occurs when the silver halide grains in a film emulsion are developed following an exposure

**C.** 'True' fog is more likely to occur with the use of slow films

**D.** Increase in the thickness of a part being irradiated results in an increase in the amount of scatter radiation produced

**E.** It is acceptable for the beam size to be greater than the film size used

## FLUOROSCOPY

**Q 9. Regarding interlocks used in fluoroscopy**

**A.** The fluoroscopy interlock prevents screening if the filament is too hot

**B.** The preparation interlock prevents a relay from being energised if the exposure factors selected could cause tube overload

**C.** The exposure interlock prevents the exposure relay from being energised without prior initiation of the preparation circuits

**D.** The guard timer is set to operate if the exposure time exceeds the set time by more than 10%

**E.** Fluoroscopy is inhibited if the screening time exceeds 10 minutes

## FILMS AND SCREENS

**Q 10. Regarding subtraction techniques**

**A.** In photographic subtraction, the mask image is produced by using a single emulsion film with a gamma of $-2$

**B.** In photographic subtraction the initial mask is known as positive mask

**C.** In digital subtraction the image used as a mask is electronically subtracted from a subsequent image

**D.** In digital subtraction it is essential to achieve almost perfect registration between initial and post-contrast images

**E.** In a digital system, the electronic signals are fed into a digital to analogue converter from where they can then be manipulated

**Q 11. The following window levels and window widths would be appropriate for the associated investigation**

**A.** Abdomen : window level (WL) 60, window width (WW) 400

**B.** Lung: WL −600, WW 1,600

**C.** Bone: WL 800, WW 2,000

**D.** Posterior Fossa : WL 35, WW 150

**E.** Brain : WL 35, WW 85

## X-RAY INTERACTIONS

**Q 12. Regarding the attenuation of monochromatic radiation**

**A.** Decreases the mean energy of the beam

**B.** Is the fractional reduction in intensity as it traverses an absorber

**C.** Is exponential

**D.** Is contributed to by photon absorption

**E.** Is contributed to by photon scatter

## X-RAY TUBES

**Q 13. The following are true**

**A.** In an X-ray tube, most of the energy of the filament electrons goes to produce X-rays

**B.** A photoelectron has the same energy as an incident X-ray photon

**C.** Characteristic K radiation is produced by electrons with energy greater than that of the K absorption edge

**D.** The output of an X-ray tube is proportional to the mAs on the control panel

**E.** The output of an X-ray tube is independent of whether the rectification is half-wave or full-wave

## IMAGE QUALITY

**Q 14. Secondary radiation grids**

A. Grid ratio equals the ratio of – [height of the lead strips] : [width of the lead strips in the grid]

B. A typical grid ratio used in most diagnostic radiology is 20 : 1

C. High-ratio grids are preferable at high kV and with very large field areas

D. Contrast improvement factor is defined as the ratio of – [contrast obtained with a grid] : [contrast obtained without a grid]

E. Bucky factor is defined as the ratio of – [exposure necessary with a grid] : [exposure necessary without a grid]

## FILMS AND SCREENS

**Q 15. The following statements regarding image quality are true**

A. Contrast between adjacent areas of a film is due to the difference in their optical densities

B. Radiographic contrast is defined as the ratio of [film gamma] : [subject contrast]

C. Screen unsharpness is greatest when using thinner screens

D. Screen unsharpness can be reduced by using coarser crystals

E. A high definition screen may typically have an intensification factor of 100

## FLUOROSCOPY

**Q 16. Regarding the image intensifier**

A. Zinc cadmium sulphide (ZnCdS) is usually used as the input phosphor

B. Caesium iodide (CsI) is usually used as the output phosphor

C. The input phosphor absorbs about 20% of the X-ray energy converting it into light

D. Photo-electrons produced in the image intensifier are accelerated by a potential difference of 25–35 V between the input and output screens

E. CsI crystals have a higher packing density than ZnCdS crystals resulting in increased screen efficiency

# FILMS AND SCREENS

**Q 17. Rare earth screens**

    **A.** Allow a lower tube loading
    **B.** Allow the use of smaller focal spots
    **C.** Produce less movement blur
    **D.** Produce less geometric distortion
    **E.** Reduce quantum mottle

# X-RAY INTERACTIONS

**Q 18. Regarding the photoelectric effect**

    **A.** Both 'free' and 'bound' electrons are involved
    **B.** Is greater in aluminium than in lead for a given photon energy
    **C.** Results in the emission of characteristic radiation
    **D.** A positron may be emitted
    **E.** Produces significant scatter radiation in the diagnostic energy range

# X-RAY TUBES

**Q 19. Regarding the X-ray tube and X-ray production**

    **A.** The focusing cup of the cathode is designed so as to concentrate the electrons on the focal spot
    **B.** A tungsten rhenium target is tougher and less likely to crack due to heating than a target made of tungsten alone
    **C.** A dual focus tube has two filaments of differing sizes which enables the production of two different sizes of focal spot
    **D.** The tube current is measured in volts
    **E.** A rotating anode tube has a significantly higher rating than a tube which has a stationary anode

# RADIATION PROTECTION

**Q 20. Regarding stochastic effects**

    **A.** The severity of the effect increases with dose
    **B.** They may be induced by very small doses of radiation
    **C.** They are typically cancers

**D.** They are of less concern with children

**E.** They have a threshold dose

## RADIATION PROTECTION

Q 21. **Regarding TLDs**

    **A.** They can only be used once

    **B.** Have a wide dose range

    **C.** Are cheap

    **D.** Lithium iodide is a suitable material

    **E.** Are relatively bulky

## RADIATION PROTECTION

Q 22. **According to the Ionising Radiation Regulations 1999**

    **A.** Only classified workers are allowed in controlled areas

    **B.** A classified worker is one who is likely to receive more than 3% of any annual dose limit

    **C.** It is the employer's responsibility to ensure that protective equipment is used by their radiation workers

    **D.** Employers are responsible for ensuring that their workers are adequately trained

    **E.** Female radiation workers are not obliged to inform their employer if they become pregnant

## RADIATION PROTECTION

Q 23. **Regarding dose limits**

    **A.** The equivalent dose for the abdomen of a woman of reproductive capacity is 13 mSv in any year

    **B.** If a worker is exposed to an effective dose greater than 20 mSv in a year the executive needs to be notified

    **C.** For a trainee under 18 years, the equivalent eye dose limit is 50 mSv in a year

    **D.** The annual equivalent dose limit to the ankle of an employee older than 18 years is 150 mSv

    **E.** The annual effective dose limit for a visitor can never exceed 1 mSv

**Q 24. Regarding tissue damage from ionising radiation**

    **A.** The greater the energy of an X-ray, the less the interaction with tissue

    **B.** The majority of tissue damage is by direct interaction of the ionising radiation

    **C.** Indirect damage is via the formation of free radicals

    **D.** Alpha and beta radiation do not cause tissue damage

    **E.** Tissue recovery does not occur

## RADIATION PROTECTION

**Q 25. The following decrease patient dose**

    **A.** Using an air gap

    **B.** Decreasing the focus-skin distance

    **C.** Coning

    **D.** Using compression

    **E.** Increasing the frame rate during fluoroscopy

Exam 7

Questions

**A 1.** **A.** true  **B.** true  **C.** false  **D.** false  **E.** false

The use of a grid decreases the amount of scatter reaching the film.
The air-gap technique achieves its effect by virtue of scattered
photons simply missing the film.
At lower kV there tends to be more side scatter production and
less scatter in a forward direction.

Farr, Allisy-Roberts. *Physics for Medical Imaging*, 1st Edn. W. B. Saunders Co.
Ltd.

**A 2.** **A.** true  **B.** true  **C.** true  **D.** true  **E.** true

Farr, Allisy-Roberts. *Physics for Medical Imaging*, 1st Edn. W. B. Saunders
Co. Ltd.

**A 3.** **A.** false  **B.** false  **C.** true  **D.** false  **E.** true

A filter is relatively transparent to its own characteristic radiation.
The filter serves to remove most of the continuous spectrum.
A single rear screen is used.
Compression is vital in order to immobilise the breast, and also to
decrease the object to film distance thus decreasing geometric
unsharpness.

Farr, Allisy-Roberts. *Physics for Medical Imaging*, 1st Edn. W. B. Saunders
Co. Ltd.

**A 4.** **A.** true  **B.** false  **C.** true  **D.** true  **E.** true

The image is affected by screen unsharpness and consequently
has a lower resolution compared to film exposed directly.
Film contrast is increased because screens diminish the effect of
scatter when compared to film exposed alone.

Curry, Thomas. *Christensen's Physics of Diagnostic Radiology*, 4th Edn.
Williams & Wilkins (Europe) Ltd.

Curry, Thomas. *Christensen's Physics of Diagnostic Radiology*, 4th Edn.
Williams & Wilkins (Europe) Ltd.

**A** **6.**   **A.** true   **B.** true   **C.** true   **D.** false   **E.** false

Alpha emission is particulate emission from radioactive decay.
The energy of electromagnetic radiation is inversely
proportional to its wavelength and derived from the equation
$E = hc/\lambda$.

Curry, Thomas. *Christensen's Physics of Diagnostic Radiology*, 4th Edn.
Williams & Wilkins (Europe) Ltd.

**A** **7.**   **A.** true   **B.** true   **C.** true   **D.** false   **E.** false

The tube rating tends to increase with increase in focal spot size.
Three-phase generators are about 35% more efficient than
single-phase generators. Thus the tube rating for a three-phase
unit is equal to $1.35 \times kV \times mA \times seconds$.

Curry, Thomas. *Christensen's Physics of Diagnostic Radiology*, 4th Edn.
Williams & Wilkins (Europe) Ltd.

**A** **8.**   **A.** true   **B.** false   **C.** false   **D.** true   **E.** false

An optical density of 0.04 equates to a difference in light
transmission of 10%.
'True' fog occurs when the silver halide grains in an emulsion are
developed in the absence of exposure to light or X-rays.
'True' fog is more likely to be seen with the use of high-speed
films due to their highly sensitised grains.
It is good radiological practice for the beam size to be less than
the film size used, and as such evidence of collimation should be
seen on every exposed film.

Armstrong. *Lecture Notes on the Physics of radiology*, 1st Edn. Clinical Press
Ltd., 1990.

**A** **9.**   **A.** true   **B.** true   **C.** true   **D.** false   **E.** true

The guard timer terminates an exposure if the exposure time
exceeds the set time by 1%.

Exam 7

Answers

By UK law fluoroscopy is inhibited if screening time exceeds 10 minutes. In practice there is a 5 minutes reminder.

Armstrong. *Lecture Notes on the Physics of Radiology*, 1st Edn. Clinical Press Ltd., 1990.

**A** **10.** **A.** false **B.** true **C.** true **D.** true **E.** false

The single emulsion used for the mask image has a gamma of −1.
It is known as a positive mask because if it is superimposed on the original radiograph all the information is 'masked out'.
The electronic signals are fed into an analogue to digital converter to produce digital signals which are then manipulated.

Armstrong. *Lecture Notes on the Physics of Radiology*, 1st Edn. Clinical Press Ltd., 1990.

**A** **11.** **A.** true **B.** true **C.** true **D.** true **E.** true

These values are used in a CT unit in my department. They are essentially appropriate for the investigations described but the values in your department may differ slightly.

**A** **12.** **A.** false **B.** true **C.** true **D.** true **E.** true

Attenuation of a monochromatic beam by an absorber does not change the quality of the beam but reduces the number of photons in the beam i.e. there is a decrease in quantity of photons.

Curry, Thomas. *Christensen's Physics of Diagnostic Radiology*, 4th Edn. Williams & Wilkins (Europe) Ltd.

**A** **13.** **A.** false **B.** false **C.** true **D.** true **E.** false

Only 1% of the energy of electrons goes to produce X-rays. The rest is liberated as heat.
A photoelectron has less energy than the incident photon.
Tube loading is 35% more efficient with full-wave rectification.

Armstrong. *Lecture Notes on the Physics of Radiology*, 1st Edn. Clinical Press Ltd.

**14.** **A.** false **B.** false **C.** true **D.** true **E.** false

Grid ratio is a ratio of the height of the lead strips to the distance between them.
A typical grid ratio is 8:1.
High-ratio grids are preferable at high kV and with very large field areas because more scatter is produced in this setting.
The ratio of exposure necessary with a grid to that without a grid describes grid factor. Bucky factor = incident radiation: transmitted radiation.

Farr, Allisy-Roberts. *Physics for Medical Imaging*, 1st Edn. W. B. Saunders Co. Ltd.

**15.** **A.** true **B.** false **C.** false **D.** false **E.** false

Radiographic contrast = film gamma × subject contrast.
Screen unsharpness is greatest for thicker screens.
Screen unsharpness is reduced with screens composed of fine crystals.
A high definition screen or 'detail' screen typically has an intensification factor of 35.

Farr, Allisy-Roberts. *Physics for Medical Imaging*, 1st Edn. W. B. Saunders Co. Ltd.

**16.** **A.** false **B.** false **C.** false **D.** false **E.** true

CsI is usually used as the input phosphor.
ZnCdS is usually used as the output phosphor.
The input phosphor absorbs about 60% of the X-ray energy.
A potential difference of 25–35 kV is applied between the input and output phosphors.
CsI has needle-like crystals which can be aligned and packed tightly together.

Farr, Allisy-Roberts. *Physics for Medical Imaging*, 1st Edn. W. B. Saunders Co. Ltd.

**17.** **A.** true **B.** true **C.** true **D.** true **E.** false

As lower exposures are required with fast-film screen systems, the use of rarer screens can lead to problems with noise.

Curry, Thomas. *Christensen's Physics of Diagnostic Radiology*, 4th Edn. Williams & Wilkins (Europe) Ltd.

Exam 7

Answers

**A** **18.** **A.** false **B.** false **C.** true **D.** false **E.** false

The photoelectric effect involves an interaction with a bound electron.
A positron is emitted in pair production.
Most scatter in diagnostic radiology is produced by the Compton process. However, when contrast agents such as barium and iodine are used, secondary radiation via the photoelectric effect may reach the film.

Curry, Thomas. *Christensen's Physics of Diagnostic Radiology*, 4th Edn. Williams & Wilkins (Europe) Ltd.

**A** **19.** **A.** true **B.** true **C.** true **D.** false **E.** true

The tube current is measured in mAs.

Curry, Thomas. *Christensen's Physics of Diagnostic Radiology*, 4th Edn. Williams & Wilkins (Europe) Ltd.

**A** **20.** **A.** false **B.** true **C.** true **D.** false **E.** false

The probability of a stochastic effect occurring increases with dose, not the severity of the effect, and thus these effects may be induced by very small doses of radiation.
Children are believed to be more radiosensitive than adults and have a longer life in which to express any cancer.
Deterministic effects have threshold doses.

Farr, Allisy-Roberts. *Physics for Medical Imaging*, 1st Edn. W. B. Saunders Co. Ltd.

**A** **21.** **A.** false **B.** true **C.** false **D.** false **E.** false

TLDs (thermoluminescent dosimeters) are relatively expensive, small, can be re-used and react to a wide range of dose (0.1–2,000 mSv).
Lithium fluoride is a common material for TLDs.

Farr, Allisy-Roberts. *Physics for Medical Imaging*, 1st Edn. W. B. Saunders Co. Ltd.

**A** **22.** **A.** false **B.** false **C.** false **D.** true **E.** true

A classified worker is one who is likely to receive more than 30% of any annual dose limit.

Radiation workers are themselves responsible and obliged to use available protective equipment.

*Ionising Radiation Regulations 1999.*

**A 23. A.** false **B.** true **C.** true **D.** false **E.** false

The equivalent dose for the abdomen of a woman of reproductive capacity is 13 mSv in consecutive period of THREE months.
The limit on equivalent dose for the hands, forearms, feet and ankles shall be 500 mSv in a calendar year for an employee 18 years and older.
If a person is exposed to ionising radiation resulting from the medical exposure of another, the limit on effective dose for any such person shall be 5 mSv in any period of 5 consecutive calendar years, which may be greater than 1 mSv per year.

*Ionising Radiation Regulations 1999.*

**A 24. A.** true **B.** true **C.** true **D.** false **E.** false

Alpha, beta and gamma radiation, X-rays and electrons are all examples of ionising radiation.
Tissue can recover from damage by ionising radiation, although this depends on dose and frequency of exposure.

Farr, Allisy-Roberts. *Physics for Medical Imaging*, 1st Edn. W. B. Saunders Co. Ltd.

**A 25. A.** false **B.** false **C.** true **D.** true **E.** false

An air gap increases patient dose, along with contrast.
Increasing the focus skin distance decreases patient dose.
Decreasing the fluoroscopy frame decreases patient dose.

Farr, Allisy-Roberts. *Physics for Medical Imaging*, 1st Edn. W. B. Saunders Co. Ltd.

## RADIOACTIVITY

**Q 1.** **The following are true of alpha particles**

  A. They are identical to helium nuclei
  B. They travel relatively quickly through matter
  C. They produce a relatively small amount of ionisation per unit length of track
  D. They tend to travel only short distances in solid material
  E. They serve no useful purpose in diagnostic radiography

## IMAGE QUALITY

**Q 2.** **Regarding grids and grid cut-off**

  A. Lateral decentring produces a radiograph that is light on one side and dark on the other side
  B. Focus grid distance decentring produces a uniformly light radiograph
  C. Combined lateral and focus grid distance decentring produces a radiograph that is light at the periphery
  D. Combined lateral and focus grid distance decentring is the commonest type of grid of cut-off encountered in every day practice
  E. Moving grids incur an increased patient radiation dose compared to static grids

## TOMOGRAPHY

**Q 3.** **Regarding tomography**

  A. Wide-angle tomography is also known as zonography
  B. The use of wide-angle tomography would be effective for imaging the inner ear
  C. Narrow-angle tomography is useful for imaging tissues with a lot of natural contrast

**D.** Phantom images tend to be produced more frequently in narrow-angle tomography

**E.** Narrow-angle tomography achieves its effects by utilising maximal blurring of obscuring shadows

# GAMMA IMAGING

**Q 4. Concerning the isotopes of iodine**

**A.** I-123 has a half-life of 13 days

**B.** I-131 has a half-life of 8 days

**C.** I-125 is a beta emitter

**D.** A low-energy general-purpose collimator is used with I-123

**E.** A high-energy general-purpose collimator is used with I-131

# FILMS AND SCREENS

**Q 5. Radiographic contrast depends upon**

**A.** Inherent film contrast

**B.** Film fog

**C.** Scatter radiation

**D.** Subject contrast

**E.** Conditions under which the film is developed

# X-RAY INTERACTIONS

**Q 6. Regarding the linear attenuation coefficient (LAC)**

**A.** Of tissue, is dependent on the density of the tissue

**B.** For monochromatic radiation the LAC is inversely proportional to the half-value layer of the tissue

**C.** Of an absorber, is greater for a high-energy beam than it is for a low-energy beam

**D.** Of fat, is greater than the LAC of muscle within the diagnostic energy range

**E.** Has units – per metre

# X-RAY TUBES

**Q 7. Regarding the production of X-rays**

**A.** Tungsten may be used as the material in either the cathode or the anode

**B.** Tungsten is used as the target material primarily due to its high thermal conductivity

C. The mA is controlled by varying the filament temperature

D. The quality of an X-ray beam depends upon the square of the kVp, mAs, atomic number and waveform

E. X-ray production is 99% efficient

## FILMS AND SCREENS

**Q 8.** **The following statements are true**

A. Total unsharpness = square root of [geometric unsharpness squared + movement unsharpness squared + screen unsharpness squared]

B. Minimum total unsharpness occurs when the individual blurrings are nearly equal

C. Signal to noise ratio (SNR) is reduced when a large number of X-ray photons are absorbed by a screen

D. The use of screens decreases noise

E. Using a higher kV reduces SNR

## CT

**Q 9.** **Computed Tomography (CT)**

A. Back projection is more effective than filtered back projection at reducing the blurring at edges of an image

B. Partial volume effects are reduced by using both a large slice thickness and large pixel size

C. Soft tissues, excluding fat, only cover a range of about 80 CT numbers

D. The effect of beam hardening is the progressive reduction in the CT number of an individual tissue as it is traversed by the X-ray beam

E. 'Bow tie' filters are used to compensate for the diminishing patient thickness towards the edges of the fan beam

## GAMMA IMAGING

**Q 10.** **The following statements are true**

A. In gamma imaging, spatial resolution (SR) can be calculated from the full width at half maximum (FWHM) of a line source

B. The intrinsic resolution of a gamma camera is 1–2 mm

**C.** Linearity of a gamma camera can be assessed by imaging a flood field source

**D.** Energy resolution of a gamma camera is typically 25% of the peak energy

**E.** The better the energy resolution of a gamma camera, the better its spatial resolution

# FILMS AND SCREENS

**Q 11. The effects of quantum mottle are reduced by the following**

**A.** When image contrast is high

**B.** When imaging larger objects

**C.** By increasing the window width of a digital image

**D.** By the use of frame averaging in digital subtraction techniques

**E.** By increasing the kVp when using a film screen combination

# X-RAY INTERACTIONS AND FILTERS

**Q 12. Regarding X-ray filters**

**A.** Aluminium and copper are the materials of choice in a compound filter

**B.** In a compound filter the lower atomic number filter faces the X-ray tube

**C.** Characteristic radiation produced in the aluminium filter significantly adds to patient skin dose

**D.** Filtration is the process of decreasing the mean energy of polychromatic radiation by passing it through an absorber

**E.** The copper in a compound filter is better for dealing with low-energy radiation

# X-RAY TUBES

**Q 13. Regarding the production of X-rays**

**A.** Materials of higher atomic number are more efficient X-ray producers

**B.** Higher energy characteristic radiation is produced with higher atomic number elements

**C.** The quality of an X-ray beam depends on the square of the kVp

**D.** The quantity of X-rays produced depends on the mAs

**E.** Tungsten is commonly used as the anode target material due to its high vapour pressure

## IMAGE QUALITY

**Q 14. Regarding the modulation transfer function (MTF)**

**A.** The MTF is calculated from the line spread function by Fourier transformation

**B.** The total MTF of a complete imaging system is obtained by adding the individual MTFs of each component

**C.** The frequency of line pairs per millimetre giving a 10% response on the MTF curve defines the resolving power of an imaging system

**D.** The maximum value of MTF is normally less than 1

**E.** MTF is proportional to the ratio of information recorded to the information available

## TOMOGRAPHY

**Q 15. Regarding simultaneous multi-plane tomography**

**A.** Several layers of X-ray film are all exposed simultaneously during a single tomographic sweep

**B.** Intensifying screens, of increasing speed, are used between each successive layer of film

**C.** The reduction in patient dose by using this technique compared to single-film tomography is approximately 90%

**D.** The image quality produced is on par with that of single-film tomography

**E.** The several layers of X-ray film are placed in a special 'book cassette' prior to exposure

## RADIOACTIVITY

**Q 16. Iodine-131 has a half-life of 8 days. Its activity at 9 am on 1st March was 44.4 MBq. Which of the following statements are true regarding the activity after time n, where n equals a number of half-lives?**

**A.** Activity can be calculated from the formula $A^n = A^o$ divided by $(2^n)$, where $A^n$ = decayed activity and $A^o$ = initial activity

**B.** Its activity at 9 am on 25th March will be 15.5 MBq

**C.** Its activity at 9 am on 25th March will be 11.1 MBq

**D.** Its activity at 9 am on 25th March will be 5.55 MBq

**E.** Its activity at 9 am on 25th March cannot be calculated from the amount of information given

# X-RAY INTERACTIONS

**Q 17. Regarding interactions of X-rays with matter**

**A.** Attenuation = absorption + scatter

**B.** Half-value layer (HVL) is a measure of the penetrating power of an X-ray beam

**C.** 10 HVLs reduces the intensity of an X-ray beam by a factor of 10

**D.** Linear attenuation coefficient (LAC) increases as the density of the absorber material increases

**E.** HVL increases as the density of the absorber increases

# IMAGE QUALITY

**Q 18. Secondary radiation grids**

**A.** Grid cut-off is greatest with both high-ratio grids and short grid focus distances

**B.** With a focused grid, about 50% of the primary radiation is attenuated by the edges of the lead strips

**C.** Lateral grid decentring produces a uniformly dark film

**D.** Combined lateral and focus-grid distance decentring produces a radiograph that is light on one side and dark on the other

**E.** Grids are routinely used when X-raying children

# X-RAY TUBES

**Q 19. The following are true regarding an X-ray tube**

**A.** At the target of an X-ray tube, the effective 'focal area' is smaller than the actual 'focal area'

**B.** The target angle is commonly 6–20 degrees

**C.** An X-ray tube for most diagnostic imaging has 2 filaments and 2 focal spots of differing sizes

**D.** The effective 'focal spot' may be measured with a STAR test tool

**E.** Blooming of a focal spot occurs particularly at low kV values and with small focal spots

Exam 8

Questions

# RADIATION PROTECTION

**Q 20. According to the IR(ME)R 2000 regulations the employer**

  **A.** Classifies workers

  **B.** Writes local rules

  **C.** Ensures employees are properly trained

  **D.** Must justify each radiation exposure

  **E.** Must ensure that a medical physics expert is involved, to some degree, in every medical exposure

# RADIATION PROTECTION

**Q 21. The following are typical effective doses**

  **A.** Chest X-ray 1 mSv

  **B.** Barium enema 9 mSv

  **C.** IVU 1 mSv

  **D.** Nuclear medicine cardiac imaging (99 m Tc) 6 mSv

  **E.** Nuclear medicine lung ventilation (81 m Kr) 1 mSv

# RADIATION PROTECTION

**Q 22. Regarding radiation protection**

  **A.** A 0.25 mm lead equivalent apron should stop 90% of the direct output of an X-ray tube

  **B.** Portable X-ray machines must allow the operator to stand at least 1 m away

  **C.** The simplest form of radiation protection comes from using the inverse square law

  **D.** 1 mm of lead is equivalent to 120 cm of concrete

  **E.** Lead aprons should be worn when involved in nuclear medicine

# RADIATION PROTECTION

**Q 23. Regarding designated areas**

  **A.** A controlled area is where a person is likely to receive an effective dose greater than 6 mSv per year

  **B.** A supervised area is where a person is likely to receive an effective dose greater than 1 mGy per year

  **C.** Anyone entering a controlled area must be able to demonstrate that their dose falls within the dose limits

**D.** Records regarding radiation equipment used within a controlled area must be kept for a minimum of 5 years

**E.** Only a classified worker can enter a controlled area

## RADIATION PROTECTION

**Q 24. According to IR(ME)R 2000**

**A.** The referrer is responsible for justification of a medical exposure

**B.** Only a practitioner can authorise a medical exposure

**C.** It is up to the referrer to supply enough medical information to justify a medical exposure

**D.** The practitioner can never be the referrer

**E.** The must be a net benefit for a medical exposure to take place

## RADIATION PROTECTION

**Q 25. IR(ME)R 2000 contains the following to ensure optimisation of medical exposures**

**A.** A dose as low as reasonably practicable (ALARP)

**B.** Direct screen fluoroscopy

**C.** Use of diagnostic reference levels is required

**D.** Routine quality assurance is not required

**E.** Clinical evaluation of outcome is required

Exam 8

Questions

**A 1.** **A.** true  **B.** false  **C.** false  **D.** true  **E.** true

Alpha particles have a relatively large mass and this together with their double charge means that they travel relatively slowly through matter and produce a large amount of ionisation per unit length of track.

Armstrong. *Lecture Notes on the physics of Radiology,* 1st Edn. Clinical Press Ltd., 1990.

**A 2.** **A.** false  **B.** false  **C.** false  **D.** true  **E.** true

Lateral decentring produces a uniformly light radiograph.
Focus grid distance decentring produces a film which is light at the periphery.
Combined lateral and focus grid distance decentring produces a radiograph that is light on one side and dark on the other.
There is an increased patient dose incurred with moving grids due to the inevitable lateral decentring that occurs resulting in primary radiation losses of up to 20%.

Armstrong, *Lecture Notes on the Physics of Radiology,* 1st Edn. Clinical Press Ltd., 1990.

**A 3.** **A.** false  **B.** true  **C.** false  **D.** true  **E.** false

Narrow-angle tomography is otherwise known as zonography. Wide-angle tomography is most effective in studying tissues that have a lot of natural contrast i.e. the inner ear. Conversely narrow-angled tomography is useful for imaging tissues with low natural contrast, i.e. the kidneys.
A phantom image may occur as a result of the superimposition of the blur margins of regularly recurring structures.
Alternatively, they may also be produced by the displacement of the blur margins of dense objects which then simulate less dense objects.

Narrow-angled tomography uses a narrow arc and aims to see the whole of a particular structure, undistorted and sharply defined. It is wide-angled tomography that utilises maximal blurring.

Armstrong. *Lecture Notes on the Physics of Radiology,* 1st Edn. Clinical Press Ltd., 1990.

**A** **4.**   **A.** false   **B.** true   **C.** false   **D.** true   **E.** true

I-123 has a half-life of 13 hours.
I-125 is a gamma emitter.
I-123 emits a gamma ray with an energy of 159 keV.
I-131 emits gamma rays with energies of 80, 204 and 364 keV.

Re.: Curry, Thomas. *Christensen's Physics of Diagnostic Radiology,* 4th Edn. Williams & Wilkins (Europe) Ltd.

**A** **5.**   **A.** true   **B.** true   **C.** true   **D.** true   **E.** true

Inherent film contrast is determined by the size and distribution of the grains of silver halide produced in the manufacturing process.
Film fog, in turn, is determined by the way the film is stored and its developing conditions.
Subject contrast is influenced by several factors such as kV, scatter radiation, differences in patient thickness, differences in density and atomic number.
The way a film is stored and the conditions under which it is developed have an effect on film fog.

Armstrong. *Lecture Notes on the Physics of Radiology,* 1st Edn. Clinical Press Ltd.

**A** **6.**   **A.** true   **B.** true   **C.** false   **D.** false   **E.** true

A high-energy beam is more penetrating than a low-energy beam. Hence, an absorber is less efficient at attenuating at high energies.
Muscle has a greater physical density than fat and consequently has a higher linear attenuation coefficient.

Curry, Thomas. *Christensen's Physics of Diagnostic Radiology,* 4th Edn. Williams & Wilkins (Europe) Ltd.

**A 7.** **A.** true **B.** false **C.** true **D.** false **E.** false

W is chosen as the target material because of its high Z, high melting point and low vapour pressure.
The square of the kVp, mAs, atomic number and waveform determine the number of X-rays produced i.e. the quantity.
X-ray production is 1% efficient. 99% of the incident energy goes into heat production.

Farr, Allisy-Roberts. *Physics for Medical Imaging,* 1st Edn. W. B. Saunders Co. Ltd.

**A 8.** **A.** true **B.** true **C.** false **D.** false **E.** true

SNR increases with an increasing number of X-ray photons absorbed.
The use of screens increases noise.
However, a higher kV also incurs less dose to the patient.

Farr, Allisy-Roberts. *Physics for Medical Imaging,* 1st Edn. W. B. Saunders Co. Ltd.

**A 9.** **A.** false **B.** false **C.** true **D.** true **E.** true

Filtered back projection is more effective at reducing the blurring at edges of an image.
Both thinner slices and smaller pixels should be used to reduce partial volume artefacts. Thus making it more likely that high-contrast objects are contained within their own voxel, and do not increase the average CT number of neighbouring voxels.

Farr, Allisy-Roberts. *Physics for Medical Imaging,* 1st Edn. W. B. Saunders Co. Ltd.

**A 10.** **A.** true **B.** true **C.** false **D.** false **E.** true

Imaging a line source provides a line spread function from which FWHM is calculated.
Linearity is assessed by imaging a line source.
Energy resolution is the ability to distinguish between separate gamma rays of differing energies. It is typically 12% of the peak energy.

With improved energy resolution there is better resolution of scatter resulting in improved spatial resolution.

Farr, Allisy-Roberts. *Physics for Medical Imaging,* 1st Edn. W. B. Saunders Co. Ltd.

**A** **11.** **A.** true   **B.** true   **C.** false   **D.** true   **E.** false

A narrow window width increases image contrast.
When using a higher kVp with a film screen combination, the intensification factor of the screen is increased. As a consequence the number of photons required to produce an image is reduced. This results in increased quantum mottle.

Curry, Thomas. *Christensen's Physics of Diagnostic Radiology,* 4th Edn. Williams & Wilkins (Europe) Ltd.

**A** **12.** **A.** true   **B.** false   **C.** false   **D.** false   **E.** false

When using a compound filter the higher atomic number material filter (copper) faces the X-ray tube and the lower atomic number material filter (aluminium) faces the patient. The purpose of the lower atomic number material is to absorb any characteristic radiation produced in the higher atomic number material.
The characteristic radiation produced by the aluminium filter has only a very low energy (1.5 keV) and is absorbed in the air gap between the patient and the filter.
Filtration increases the mean energy of polychromatic radiation. Copper is better for dealing with high-energy radiation.

Curry, Thomas. *Christensen's Physics of Diagnostic Radiology,* 4th Edn. Williams & Wilkins (Europe) Ltd.

**A** **13.** **A.** true   **B.** true   **C.** false   **D.** true   **E.** false

The nature of the target material also determines the energy of the characteristic radiation produced. This is higher for higher atomic number elements.
The quality of X-rays depends upon kVp and the waveform.
The quantity of X-rays produced depends on the mAs, atomic number, square of the kVp and the waveform.

Tungsten has a low vapour pressure in association with a high melting point.

Armstrong. *Lecture Notes on the Physics of Radiology,* 1st Edn. Clinical Press Ltd., 1990.

**A 14. A.** true **B.** false **C.** true **D.** true **E.** true

The MTF of a complete system is a product of the individual MTFs of each component.
Whilst the MTF is normally less than 1, in xeroradiography values slightly greater than 1 (e.g. 1.1) may be obtained. This is due to the special property in xeroradiography known as edge enhancement.

Armstrong. *Lecture Notes on the Physics of Radiology,* 1st Edn. Clinical Press Ltd., 1990.

**A 15. A.** true **B.** true **C.** false **D.** false **E.** true

The screens of increasing speed are to allow for the attenuation caused by the reducing intensity of X-rays as they pass through successive layers.
The reduction in patient dose is not as great as might be anticipated. Overall there is an exposure dose per film of about 50% that of single-film techniques.
This technique results in poor-quality tomograms. This is due to the uncontrolled scatter radiation produced which impairs film quality.

Armstrong. *Lecture Notes on the Physics of Radiology,* 1st Edn. Clinical Press Ltd., 1990.

**A 16. A.** true **B.** false **C.** false **D.** true **E.** false

Curry, Thomas. *Christensen's Physics of Diagnostic Radiology,* 4th Edn. Williams & Wilkins (Europe) Ltd.

**A 17. A.** true **B.** true **C.** false **D.** true **E.** false

10 HVLs would reduce the intensity by 2 factor 10 i.e. 1000.
As the density of the absorbing material increases the HVL decreases. HVL is inversely proportional to LAC.

Farr, Allisy-Roberts. *Physics for Medical Imaging,* 1st Edn. W. B. Saunders Co. Ltd.

**A** **18.** **A.** true  **B.** false  **C.** false  **D.** true  **E.** false

20% of the primary radiation is attenuated by the edges of the lead strips.
Lateral grid decentring produces a uniformly light film.
Grids are also not used with thin body parts.

Farr, Allisy-Roberts. *Physics for Medical Imaging,* 1st Edn. W. B. Saunders Co. Ltd.

**A** **19.** **A.** true  **B.** true  **C.** true  **D.** true  **E.** true

Blooming also tends to occur when the tube is operated at high mA as focusing is less precise.

Farr, Allisy-Roberts. *Physics for Medical Imaging,* 1st Edn. W. B. Saunders Co. Ltd.

**A** **20.** **A.** true  **B.** true  **C.** true  **D.** false  **E.** true

The practitioner must justify each radiation exposure.

*IR(ME)R 2000.*

**A** **21.** **A.** false  **B.** true  **C.** false  **D.** true  **E.** false

CXR 0.1 mSv.
IVU 5 mSv.
Lung ventilation 0.1 mSv.

Farr, Allisy-Roberts. *Physics for Medical Imaging,* 1st Edn. W. B. Saunders Co. Ltd.

**A** **22.** **A.** false  **B.** false  **C.** true  **D.** false  **E.** false

It should stop 90% of the SCATTERED output.
The operator must be able to stand 2 m away from the tube.
Using the inverse square law and increasing the distance of people from the tube/patient.
1 mm of lead is equivalent to 120 mm of concrete and 12 mm of barium plaster.
In the presence of high-energy radiation from nuclear imaging, a lead apron acts as an X-ray source, and therefore should not be used.

Farr, Allisy-Roberts. *Physics for Medical Imaging,* 1st Edn. W. B. Saunders Co. Ltd.

**A** **23.** **A.** true  **B.** false  **C.** true  **D.** false  **E.** false

Supervised area = greater than 1 mSv.
Records regarding monitoring of equipment must be kept for a minimum of 2 years.

*The Ionising Radiations Regulations 1999.*

**A** **24.** **A.** false  **B.** false  **C.** true  **D.** false  **E.** true

The practitioner is responsible for justification of a medical exposure.
An operator can authorise a medical exposure in accordance with guidelines laid down by a practitioner.
A practitioner can request a medical exposure and thus act as a referrer, fulfilling the duties and obligations of both.

*IR(ME)R 2000.*

**A** **25.** **A.** true  **B.** false  **C.** true  **D.** false  **E.** true

Only image intensification fluoroscopy is allowed.

*IR(ME)R 2000.*

## X-RAY INTERACTIONS

**Q 1.** **Which of the following interactions between X-rays and matter do not result in a change in energy of the incident photon**

- **A.** Pair production
- **B.** Photodisintegration
- **C.** Photoelectric effect
- **D.** Coherent scattering
- **E.** Compton scattering

## XERORADIOGRAPHY

**Q 2.** **In xeroradiography**

- **A.** Crystalline selenium is used
- **B.** Pure selenium must be used
- **C.** The selenium layer has a thickness of 130 $\mu$m
- **D.** Has no advantages over conventional mammography
- **E.** The developing process is dry and rapid

## X-RAY INTERACTIONS

**Q 3.** **The following are true**

- **A.** In Thompson scattering, photons are scattered with an associated change in energy
- **B.** Compton scattering depends only on the number of electrons per unit mass
- **C.** The probability of the photoelectric effect occurring increases with increasing photon energy
- **D.** The Compton effect is dependent upon the atomic number (Z) of the material irradiated
- **E.** The mass attenuation coefficient (MAC) is dependent upon both the linear attenuation coefficient (LAC) and the density of the material irradiated

## FILMS AND SCREENS

**Q 4.** **The following statements regarding the characteristic curve are true**

  A. The characteristic curve (CC) is a graph of optical density (X-axis) versus relative exposure (Y-axis)
  B. The part of the CC which relates to correct exposure is usually at the shoulder region of the curve
  C. Film gamma refers to the area under the CC
  D. In the solarisation region of the CC, increasing the exposure further produces an increase in film density
  E. Solarisation film is usually used for film copying

## FLUOROSCOPY

**Q 5.** **Regarding image quality in image intensifier (II) systems**

  A. The spatial resolution (SR) of the II alone is about 4–5 lp/mm
  B. When imaging with a 35 mm film from the II, the SR is about 2 lp/mm
  C. The SR of a TV camera system is about 1 lp/mm
  D. Veiling glare is worse with larger sizes of II
  E. A vidicon camera has a gamma of 0.8, whilst a plumbicon camera has a gamma of 1.0

## CT

**Q 6.** **Regarding image quality in CT**

  A. For high-contrast objects, the spatial resolution (SR) of a CT scanner approaches 5 lp/mm
  B. For low-contrast objects (1–2% contrast), an object may need to be 5–10 mm in diameter before it can be resolved
  C. Contrast in a structure is usually only detectable if its contrast is 10 times greater than the noise in the image
  D. Contrast resolution in CT is 0.5%
  E. 'Bone algorithms' are used to enhance spatial resolution

# RADIOACTIVITY

**Q 7.  Regarding radioactivity**

    **A.** Stable lighter radioactive nuclei contain nearly equal numbers of protons and neutrons

    **B.** Stable heavy radioactive nuclei contain a greater proportion of neutrons than protons

    **C.** Isotopes of an element are nuclides which have the same number of protons but differing number of neutrons

    **D.** Isotopes of an element are nuclides which have the same chemical properties but differing physical properties

    **E.** Isotopes of an element are nuclides which have the same position in the periodic table

# GAMMA IMAGING

**Q 8.  Regarding the half-lives of radionuclides**

    **A.** The half-life of Krypton-81 m is 13 seconds

    **B.** The half-life of Nitrogen-13 is 100 minutes

    **C.** The half-life of Carbon-11 is 200 minutes

    **D.** The half-life of Technechium-99 is 6 hours

    **E.** The half-life of Fluorine-18 is 112 minutes

# GAMMA IMAGING

**Q 9.  Regarding radionuclides and their principle uses**

    **A.** Indium-111: Tumour detection

    **B.** Galium-67: Myocardial imaging

    **C.** Galium-67: Tumour detection

    **D.** Kypton-81 m: Lung perfusion imaging

    **E.** Thalium-201: Myocardial perfusion imaging

# X-RAY TUBES

**Q 10.  The following are true regarding the equipment used in dental radiography**

    **A.** The total filtration of the beam should be equivalent to 2.5 mm aluminium for X-ray tube voltages up to and including 70 kV

    **B.** The X-ray tube voltage should not be lower than 50 kV and for intra-oral radiography should be preferably about 70 kV

**C.** The X-ray assembly should be marked to identify the nominal focal spot position

**D.** When using intra-oral film, a minimum focal spot to skin distance of not less than 20 cm for equipment operating above 60 kV is required

**E.** The exposure switch should be arranged so that the operator can be at least 1 m away from the tube and the patient during exposure

## FILMS AND SCREENS

**Q 11. Regarding geometry of the X-ray image**

**A.** Sharpness is the ability of an X-ray film screen system to define an edge

**B.** Sharpness is independent of the contrast of an image

**C.** Parallax is seen with single-emulsion films

**D.** Absorption unsharpness is greatest for round or oval objects without sharp edges

**E.** Absorption unsharpness is greatest for coned-shaped objects

## DOSIMETRY

**Q 12. Regarding scintillation counters**

**A.** Sodium iodide may be used as a scintillation phosphor

**B.** Crystals of potassium iodide may be used as a scintillation phosphor

**C.** Crystals of anthracene and naphthalene may be used as scintillation phosphors

**D.** Scintillation counters cannot distinguish between radiations of different energies

**E.** A scintillation counter has both a longer dead time and a lower detection efficiency of radiation compared to Geiger Muller tubes

## X-RAY INTERACTIONS

**Q 13. Regarding subject contrast**

**A.** This refers to the difference in the intensity of transmitted radiation between one part of a subject compared to another part

**B.** The photoelectric effect is the most important contributor to subject contrast in diagnostic radiology

**C.** Higher kVp X-rays produce greater subject contrast than lower kVp X-rays

**D.** Low kVp exposures only permit a narrow exposure latitude

**E.** Contrast media do not play a role in subject contrast

# ANGIOGRAPHY

**Q 14. Regarding the apparatus required for digital subtraction angiography**

**A.** Specially designed X-ray tubes are required

**B.** The X-ray generator should be able to provide three-phase voltage pulses and 12 pulses/cycle

**C.** A focal spot of 0.3 mm is desirable

**D.** A high-quality image intensifier is needed

**E.** The X-ray tube should incorporate a high-speed rotating anode

# X-RAY TUBES

**Q 15. Regarding X-ray production**

**A.** It is the deceleration of the electrons bombarding the target that results in the production of X-rays

**B.** X-radiation is produced by the processes of Bremsstrahlung and characteristic radiation

**C.** The anode heel effect is more noticeable on large-size X-ray film

**D.** A stationary anode tube has better cooling characteristics than a rotating anode one

**E.** A lower atomic number target produces an X-ray beam of greater intensity than a higher atomic numbered target

# X-RAY TUBES

**Q 16. Regarding rotating anode tubes**

**A.** Energy efficiency is much greater than in stationary anode tubes

**B.** The tube-loading characteristics are greater as heat is generated over a focal track

**C.** The principal heat path is via radiation across the tube vacuum

D. The induction motor is situated inside the glass envelope to ensure maximum efficiency of the tube

E. The anode has a molybdenum stem backing in order to minimise heat conduction to the rotor mechanism

## IMAGE QUALITY

**Q 17. The following are criteria for attaining a radiograph of satisfactory quality**

A. The density is controlled primarily by kV

B. Contrast is controlled primarily by mA

C. Ideally there should be minimum sharpness, whilst maintaining the true outline of the image

D. Ideally there should be maximum sharpness, whilst maintaining the true outline of the image

E. Film blackness is primarily controlled by mA

## FILMS AND SCREENS

**Q 18. The following statements are true**

A. Film gamma and exposure latitude are directly related

B. High-gamma films have a narrow exposure latitude

C. The useful density range of a film is usually 0.25–2.0 above base plus fog values

D. Typically wide latitude film is needed in mammography

E. The gamma of a film depends on the average size of the crystals in the film

## FLUOROSCOPY

**Q 19. The following statements regarding fluoroscopy are true**

A. Quantum mottle is noticeable in both fluoroscopy and radiography

B. Noise reduces the perceptibility of structures having high contrast

C. For a structure to be detectable, its contrast must be at least 10 times the noise relative to the signal

D. Image quality in the less bright areas of an image is limited by noise

E. Spatial resolution improves with structures of higher contrast

# RADIATION PROTECTION

**Q 20. Regarding foetal irradiation**

- **A.** Exposure to the pregnant employee must ensure a dose of less than 0.1 mSv to the foetus for the remainder of the pregnancy
- **B.** An abdominal X-ray to a pregnant employee can expose the foetus to as much as 4 mGy
- **C.** The ten-day rule reduces the likelihood of foetal exposure
- **D.** The foetus is most sensitive to ionising radiation during the third trimester
- **E.** Foetal exposure to ionising radiation results in an IQ drop by 30 points/Sv

# RADIATION PROTECTION

**Q 21. The natural background radiation equivalent exposure for a procedure are as follows**

- **A.** Skull X-ray – 9 days
- **B.** CT chest – 4 years
- **C.** Radionuclide bone scan (Tc 99 m) – 2 years, 6 months
- **D.** IVU – 14 months
- **E.** CT head – 10 months

# RADIATION PROTECTION

**Q 22. According to IR(ME)R 2000**

- **A.** A practitioner and operator must receive at least 1 week's training before carrying out a medical exposure
- **B.** Trainees cannot carry out medical exposures
- **C.** Employers must keep an up-to-date record of all practitioners and operators
- **D.** A practitioner cannot be an employer
- **E.** Medical exposure can take place where there is no net benefit to the patient

# RADIATION PROTECTION

**Q 23. Regarding the measurement of dose**

- **A.** Absorbed dose is measured in mGy
- **B.** Equivalent dose is measured in mGy

C. Equivalent dose is absorbed dose multiplied by the tissue-weighting factor
D. The type of ionising radiation does not affect the value of the estimated absorbed dose
E. The effective dose takes into account the variable sensitivity of different organs to ionising radiation

## RADIATION PROTECTION

**Q 24. Regarding an overexposure**

A. Only the employer needs to be informed
B. The person overexposed must be informed
C. The report from an immediate investigation into the circumstances must be kept for at least 2 years
D. An employee who has received an overexposure is not required to fulfil normal dose limitations
E. A dose limitation period applies, which is 10 years

## RADIATION PROTECTION

**Q 25. The following equipment measures reduce patient dose**

A. Using a rare earth screen
B. Using film instead of digital radiography
C. Using constant potential generators
D. Using 25 mm of aluminium beam filtration for general radiography
E. Using direct-vision fluoroscopy techniques

**A 1.** **A.** false   **B.** false   **C.** false   **D.** true   **E.** false

Coherent scattering is scattering in which radiation undergoes a change in direction without a change in wavelength, and therefore no change in energy.

Armstrong. *Lecture Notes on the Physics of Radiology*, 1st Edn. Clinical Press Ltd., 1990.

**A 2.** **A.** false   **B.** true   **C.** true   **D.** false   **E.** true

Amorphous selenium is used because it has the properties of a photoconductor.
At a thickness of 130 $\mu$m, selenium shows a maximum sensitivity to X-rays in the diagnostic energy range.
Edge enhancement occurs because the toner is attracted away from the low-voltage side to the high-voltage side of any boundary resulting in a sharp change in density.

Curry, Thomas. *Christensen's Physics of Diagnostic Radiology*, 4th Edn. Williams & Wilkins (Europe) Ltd.

**A 3.** **A.** false   **B.** false   **C.** false   **D.** false   **E.** false

In Thompson scattering, radiation undergoes a change in direction without a change in wavelength, and therefore no change in energy.
Compton scattering depends on both the physical and the electron density of the material irradiated.
The probability of the photoelectric effect occurring is inversely proportional to the cube of the incident photon energy.
The probability of the Compton effect occurring is independent of Z.
The MAC is independent of the density of an absorber.

Farr, Allisy-Roberts. *Physics for Medical Imaging*, 1st Edn. W. B. Saunders Co. Ltd.

**A** **4.** **A.** false **B.** false **C.** false **D.** false **E.** true

The CC is a graph of log relative exposure (X-axis) versus optical density (Y-axis).
The region of correct exposure relates to the straight-line portion.
Film gamma relates to the maximum slope of the straight-line portion of the CC.
In the solarisation region, increasing exposure results in decreased film density.

Farr, Allisy-Roberts. *Physics for Medical Imaging*, 1st Edn. W. B. Saunders Co. Ltd.

**A** **5.** **A.** true **B.** true **C.** true **D.** true **E.** true

But note that the SR decreases for an entire II system i.e. when used with a video camera system/photospot film.
Veiling glare is due to scattering of light particularly in the output window of the image intensifier.
Despite the gamma differences of the various cameras, the gamma value of a TV monitor system can be varied, up to 2.0, so that the contrast of the system as a whole, is increased.

Farr, Allisy-Roberts. *Physics for Medical Imaging*, 1st Edn. W. B. Saunders Co. Ltd.

**A** **6.** **A.** false **B.** true **C.** false **D.** true **E.** true

High contrast objects: SR – 1 lp/mm.
Contrast needs to be 3–5 times greater than the noise in the image for it to be detectable.
Bone algorithms enhance SR at the expense of increased noise.

Farr, Allisy-Roberts. *Physics for Medical Imaging*, 1st Edn. W. B. Saunders Co. Ltd.

**A** **7.** **A.** true **B.** true **C.** true **D.** true **E.** true

Isotopes have the same atomic number but differing mass numbers.

Farr, Allisy-Roberts. *Physics for Medical Imaging*, 1st Edn. W. B. Saunders Co. Ltd.

**A.** true **B.** false **C.** false **D.** false **E.** true

The half-life of N-13 is 10 minutes.
The half-life of C-11 is 20 minutes.
The half-life of Tc-99 is 200,000 years. Tc-99 m has a half-life of
6 hours.

Farr, Allisy-Roberts. *Physics for Medical Imaging*, 1st Edn. W. B. Saunders
Co. Ltd.

**A** 9. **A.** false **B.** false **C.** true **D.** false **E.** true

Indium-111 is used to label white cells for locating infective foci.
Krypton-81 m is used for lung ventilation studies.

Farr, Allisy-Roberts. *Physics for Medical Imaging*, 1st Edn. W. B. Saunders
Co. Ltd.

**A** 10. **A.** false **B.** true **C.** true **D.** true **E.** false

The total filtration of the beam should be equivalent to 1.5 mm
aluminium for X-ray tube voltages up to and including 70 kV, and
2.5 mm aluminium, of which 1.5 mm should be permanent for X-
ray tube voltages above 70 kV.
In fact every X-ray source assembly should be marked to identify
the nominal focal spot position.
When using intra-oral film, the equipment should be provided
with a field-defining spacer cone which will ensure a minimum
focal spot to skin distance of not less than 20 cm for equipment
operating above 60 kV and not less than 10 cm for equipment
operating at lower voltages.
For dental, mobile and portable equipment, the exposure switch
should be arranged so that the operator can be at least 2 metres
away from the tube and the patient during an exposure. For
fixed equipment, the exposure switch should be located at the
control panel.

AC1/185, AC2/7, Regulation 32, Regulation 8: *IRR 88.*

**A** 11. **A.** true **B.** false **C.** false **D.** true **E.** false

Sharpness is dependent on the contrast of an image. An unsharp
edge can easily be seen if contrast is high, conversely a sharp
edge may be poorly seen if the contrast is low.

Parallax only occurs with double-emulsion films.
Absorption unsharpness is least for cone-shaped objects.

Curry, Thomas. *Christensen's Physics of Diagnostic Radiology*, 4th Edn. Williams & Wilkins (Europe) Ltd.

**A 12. A.** true   **B.** true   **C.** true   **D.** false   **E.** false

Scintillation counters are able to distinguish between radiations of different energies (unlike GM tubes).
There is less dead time and a higher detection efficiency than GM tubes.

Armstrong. *Lecture Notes on the Physics of Radiology*, 1st Edn. Clinical Press Ltd., 1990.

**A 13. A.** true   **B.** true   **C.** false   **D.** true   **E.** false

Low kVp X-rays produce greater subject contrast as more of the primary beam will be attenuated at the lower beam energies.
Contrast media are of relatively high atomic number, and therefore enhance subject contrast due to the photoelectric effect.

Armstrong. *Lecture Notes on the Physics of Radiology*, 1st Edn. Clinical Press Ltd., 1990.

**A 14. A.** false   **B.** true   **C.** false   **D.** true   **E.** true

No special tubes are required; those already in use are usually suitable.
It is undesirable to have a very small focal spot as this reduces tube loading. In addition the focal spot size in angiography is not a limiting factor to resolution. A focal spot size of 0.6 mm is adequate. 0.3 mm is usually necessary for macro-angiography. High-speed anodes are energised with three-phase mains and rotate at about 9,000 or 17,000 rpm.

Curry, Thomas. *Christensen's Physics of Diagnostic Radiology*, 4th Edn. Williams & Wilkins (Europe) Ltd.

**A 15. A.** true   **B.** true   **C.** true   **D.** false   **E.** false

The intensity of the X-ray beam produced that passes through the anode is less than that towards the cathode. Hence, with large size X-ray films the heel effect may be visible.

The rotating anode tube has better cooling characteristics as the heat is spread over a larger target area.

Higher atomic number elements are able to produce higher intensity X-ray beams. Hence tungsten, with it atomic number of 74, is an ideal target material.

Armstrong. *Lecture Notes on the Physics of Radiology*, 1st Edn. Clinical Press Ltd., 1990.

**A** **16.** **A.** false **B.** true **C.** true **D.** false **E.** true

The energy conversion between both a rotating and stationary anode tube is identical. 99% of the energy goes towards heat production and only 1% towards X-ray production.

The induction motor is situated outside the glass envelope within the insulating oil.

Curry, Thomas. *Christensen's Physics of Diagnostic Radiology*, 4th Edn. Williams & Wilkins (Europe) Ltd.

**A** **17.** **A.** true **B.** false **C.** false **D.** true **E.** true

The density, and as a consequence the contrast, is primarily controlled by kV.

Curry, Thomas. *Christensen's Physics of Diagnostic Radiology*, 4th Edn. Williams & Wilkins (Europe) Ltd.

**A** **18.** **A.** false **B.** true **C.** true **D.** false **E.** false

Film gamma and exposure latitude are inversely related.

High-gamma, narrow-latitude films are needed in mammography.

The gamma of a film depends on the range of crystal sizes.

Farr, Allisy-Roberts. *Physics for Medical Imaging*, 1st Edn. W. B. Saunders Co. Ltd.

**A** **19.** **A.** false **B.** false **C.** false **D.** true **E.** true

Noise is not noticeable in radiography.

Noise mainly affects low-contrast structures.

Contrast needs to be 2–5 times the noise relative to the signal, i.e. a 1 mm structure will be seen if its contrast is at least 5%.

Farr, Allisy-Roberts. *Physics for Medical Imaging*, 1st Edn. W. B. Saunders Co. Ltd.

**A 20. A.** false **B.** true **C.** true **D.** false **E.** true

The dose must be less than 1 mSv for the remainder of the pregnancy. The foetus is most sensitive to radiation exposure in the first 8–15 weeks of gestation.

*The Ionising Radiations Regulations 1999.*

**A 21. A.** true **B.** true **C.** false **D.** true **E.** true

Bone scan – 1.8 years.

Farr, Allisy-Roberts. *Physics for Medical Imaging*, 1st Edn. W. B. Saunders Co. Ltd.

**A 22. A.** false **B.** false **C.** true **D.** false **E.** true

A specific amount of training is not specified, just that it is adequate.
Trainees can carry out medical exposures if adequately supervised.
An employer can be a practitioner, operator or any other person.
Medical exposure can take place for research purposes where there is no net benefit to the patient.

*IR(ME)R 2000.*

**A 23. A.** true **B.** false **C.** false **D.** true **E.** true

Effective dose (Sv) = Sum (equivalent dose × tissue weighting factor).
Equivalent dose (Sv) = Absorbed dose (Gy) × radiation weighting factor.

Farr, Allisy-Roberts. *Physics for Medical Imaging*, 1st Edn. W. B. Saunders Co. Ltd.

**A.** false   **B.** false   **C.** true   **D.** false   **E.** true

The employer should inform the executive and, where the overexposure is of an employee, their appointed doctor or employed medical advisor.
As soon as practicable, reasonable steps should be taken to notify the suspected overexposure to the person affected.
The dose limitation period is as appropriate, a calendar year or the period of consecutive calendar years.

*IR(ME)R 2000.*

**A** 25. **A.** true   **B.** false   **C.** true   **D.** false   **E.** true

Digital radiography reduces patient dose.
2.5 mm of aluminium is used a beam filtration.
Digital fluoroscopy reduces dose through means of techniques such as frame capture and frame-hold.

Farr, Allisy-Roberts. *Physics for Medical Imaging*, 1st Edn. W. B. Saunders Co. Ltd.

## FILMS AND SCREENS

**Q 1.** **Regarding films and screens**

A. Rare earth screens are faster than calcium tungstate (CaW) screens

B. CaW deliver a patient dose 2–3 times lower than rare earth screens

C. Gadolinium oxysulphide screens may be used with any type of X-ray film

D. Lanthanum oxybromide may be used with ordinary X-ray film

E. The sensitivity of a film may be extended by coating the silver halide crystals with appropriate dyes

## FILMS AND SCREENS

**Q 2.** **The following statements regarding the high kV technique are true**

A. Subject contrast is high

B. Skin dose is increased

C. Dose to deeper tissues is reduced

D. Grids are less effective compared to use with lower kV techniques

E. Efficiency of X-ray production is low

## FLUOROSCOPY

**Q 3.** **Regarding the image intensifier**

A. Brightness gain is the ratio of – [brightness of the output phosphor] : [brightness of the input phosphor]

B. Overall brightness gain is typically 5,000–10,000

C. An image is intensified, magnified and inverted by an electron lens

D. Conversion factor is a ratio of – [luminescence of the output phosphor] : [input phosphor dose rate]

E. The image produced is uniformly bright and sharp

# CT

**Q 4.   Computed tomography (CT)**

A. Second-generation scanners are of the translate-rotate type
B. Third-generation scanners are of the rotate-rotate type
C. Fourth-generation scanners are of the rotate-rotate type
D. Ring artefacts are common with the fourth-generation scanner
E. Slip-ring technology has allowed the advent of helical scanning

# FILMS AND SCREENS

**Q 5.   Regarding X-ray film**

A. Silver halide is sensitive in the blue part of the visible spectrum
B. The spectral sensitivity of silver halide can be altered by adding certain light-absorbing dyes to the emulsions
C. A latent image is only produced after the film has been both exposed and developed
D. The speed of an emulsion is predominantly dependent on the grain size distribution
E. In the film emulsion there is an excess of silver bromide compared to silver iodide

# DOSIMETRY

**Q 6.   Regarding the Geiger-Muller (GM) tube**

A. Halogen gas is added to the inert gas
B. The gas is maintained at low pressure
C. The tube requires to be operated at voltages in the plateau region
D. The potential difference across the tube ranges from 200–400 volts to 900–1,500 volts
E. The GM counter is able to distinguish between different types of radiation

# X-RAY TUBES

**Q 7.   Regarding X-ray generating apparatus**

A. The kVp meter is located in the control panel
B.  The mA meter is located in the control panel

**C.** The kVp meter is incorporated into the high-voltage circuit of the X-ray generator

**D.** The mA meter is incorporated into the high-voltage circuit of the X-ray generator

**E.** The high voltage circuit of an X-ray generator consists of a single transformer

## X-RAY INTERACTIONS

Q 8. **Regarding attenuation of an X-ray beam**

**A.** This occurs solely by absorption of photons

**B.** In the attenuation of monochromatic radiation, both the number of photons in the beam and the energy of the photons are reduced

**C.** Attenuation of monochromatic radiation is exponential

**D.** Attenuation of polychromatic radiation is exponential

**E.** Attenuation of polychromatic radiation results in beam hardening

## XERORADIOGRAPHY

Q 9. **Regarding xeroradiography**

**A.** In this process the detecting medium used is the charged surface of an amorphous selenium photoconducting plate

**B.** The latent electrostatic image is developed in the same way as photographic X-ray film

**C.** Following use, the selenium plates are stored in an uncharged state prior to re-use

**D.** Xeroradiography can produce either 'positive' or 'negative' images

**E.** A xeroradiographic process has a very narrow exposure latitude when compared to conventional film screen systems

## IMAGE QUALITY

Q 10. **Regarding grids used in diagnostic radiography**

**A.** A grid with a lower grid ratio is more efficient at removing scatter radiation compared to a high-ratio grid

**B.** A high-ratio grid has a higher bucky factor

**C.** Primary transmission refers to the amount of primary radiation absorbed by the grid

**D.** Primary transmission of a grid is inversely proportionate to grid ratio

**E.** There is always some loss of the transmission in primary radiation caused by a grid

## THE ATOM

**Q 11. Regarding the structure of an atom**

**A.** The number of electrons in the M electron shell is 8

**B.** The binding energy of an M shell electron is greater than that of an L shell electron

**C.** An isotope is a substance with the same number of protons but different number of neutrons

**D.** Isotopes have identical physical properties but different chemical properties

**E.** The number of neutrons in an atom, N, is equal to $A-Z$

## X-RAY INTERACTIONS

**Q 12. Interactions of X-rays with matter**

**A.** The second half-value layer (HVL) of a material is usually less than the first HVL

**B.** The HVL of a typical diagnostic X-ray beam is 30 cm in tissue

**C.** As an X-ray beam penetrates a material, it becomes progressively more heterogeneous

**D.** The photoelectric effect results from an interaction with a free electron

**E.** Compton scattering is independent of electron density

## X-RAY TUBES

**Q 13. Tube rating**

**A.** Increases as the effective 'focal spot' size increases

**B.** Increases as the kV increases

**C.** Is greater for a high-speed anode assembly compared to a routine rotating assembly

**D.** In continuous operation fluoroscopy, rating is partly dependent on the focal spot size

**E.** Is greater for a three-phase generator compared to a single-phase generator

# IMAGE QUALITY

### Q 14. Macro-radiography

**A.** To obtain a magnified image, the focus-object distance is decreased relative to the object film distance which is increased

**B.** A very small focal spot must be used

**C.** A grid is routinely used

**D.** Usually results in reduced patient dose

**E.** Quantum mottle is not increased

# FILMS AND SCREENS

### Q 15. Regarding intensifying screens

**A.** X-ray absorption in an intensifying screen is about 30% for tungstate and 60% for rare earth screens

**B.** Screen efficiency for screens is about 50%

**C.** Screen conversion efficiency is about 20% for tungstate and 50% for rare earth screens

**D.** Increasing the conversion efficiency of a screen reduces quantum mottle

**E.** Increasing screen thickness increases quantum mottle

# FLUOROSCOPY

### Q 16. Television systems used in image intensification

**A.** The photoconducting material in the videcon tube is lead monoxide

**B.** The photoconducting material used in the plumbicon tube is lead monoxide

**C.** The image intensifier exhibits a longer 'lag' period than the TV camera tube

**D.** In cine-radiography a frame rate of greater than 16 per second is sufficient to prevent jerky motion

**E.** The dose to the patient when using 70/100 mm photospot film, is 3–5 times smaller than with full size (puck) film

## Q 17. Regarding detectors used in computed tomography (CT)

**A.** Calcium fluoride may be used as the scintillation crystals in a CT detector

**B.** Bismuth germanate may be used as the scintillation crystals in a CT detector

**C.** Ionisation chambers are more sensitive than scintillation detectors

**D.** Scintillation detectors are more stable to voltage fluctuation compared to ionisation chambers

**E.** Ionisation chambers are well suited to the fourth-generation type of CT scanners

# FILMS AND SCREENS

## Q 18. Regarding silver recovery following film processing

**A.** In the electrolytic method silver is deposited as 90–95% pure metallic silver

**B.** In the electrolytic method silver is deposited on the anode

**C.** In the electrolytic method agitation of either the cathode or the anode serves no useful purpose

**D.** In the electrolytic method it is possible to recover silver from the wash water

**E.** The metallic replacement method is a more expensive procedure than the electrolytic method

# X-RAY TUBES

## Q 19. Portable X-ray generators

**A.** A battery-powered generator uses a battery which can store a charge equivalent to 10,000 mAs

**B.** In battery-powered generators, the voltage does not fall between exposures

**C.** In battery-powered generators the output from the transformer is single-phase full-wave rectified

**D.** A capacitor discharge generator is usually used in conjunction with a field emission X-ray tube

**E.** The advantage of a capacitor discharge generator is that it can deliver a large amount of power in an extremely short time

Exam 10

Questions

# RADIATION PROTECTION

**Q 20. The following radiation weighting factors are:**

- **A.** X-rays: 1
- **B.** Electrons: 2
- **C.** Protons: 5
- **D.** Alpha particles: 10
- **E.** Neutrons: 1

# RADIATION PROTECTION

**Q 21. Regarding classified workers**

- **A.** The majority of operators are classified workers
- **B.** Individual measurement of dose is required
- **C.** Dose records must be kept
- **D.** They must be at least 16 years old
- **E.** Must be medically assessed prior to being classified

# RADIATION PROTECTION

**Q 22. According to the Ionising Radiations Regulations 1999**

- **A.** A radiation protection advisor (RPA) must be consulted regarding the requirement for controlled areas
- **B.** A radiation protection supervisor (RPS) must be consulted regarding servicing and correct use of equipment
- **C.** A RPA does not need to be consulted if the equipment does not cause a dose rate of more than $1\mu$Sv/h at a distance of 0.1 m from any accessible surface
- **D.** A RPA needs to be consulted whenever an employer plans to use a radioactive substance
- **E.** A RPS is appointed to secure compliance with the local rules

# RADIATION PROTECTION

**Q 23. The following dose limits apply**

- **A.** The annual effective dose for a trainee under 18 years of age is 6 mSv
- **B.** The annual equivalent dose limit for the skin of a member of the public is 150 mSv
- **C.** Whatever the annual dose limit, the effective dose limit for employees over 5 consecutive years is 100 mSv

**D.** The annual effective dose limit for hands of an employee is 500 mSv

**E.** The annual equivalent dose limit for hands of a member of the public is 50 mSv

## RADIATION PROTECTION

**Q 24. Regarding the damaging effects of ionising radiation**

**A.** Genetic effects are clearly identified in children of irradiated parents

**B.** Tissues undergoing regular cell division are more radiosensitive than non-dividing tissues

**C.** Deterministic effects occur due to radiation-induced cell death

**D.** The threshold dose for hair loss is 3 Gy

**E.** Deterministic effects usually have a long latent period

## RADIATION PROTECTION

**Q 25. IR(ME)R 2000**

**A.** Provides no indication as to the training required by a practitioner or operator prior to medical exposure

**B.** Regulates that employer's written procedures need to include procedures to correctly identify a patient

**C.** Regulates that patient information detailing the risks associated with ionising radiation must be given to all patients undergoing a significant medical exposure

**D.** Regulates that alternative diagnostic techniques must have been considered prior to a medical exposure

**E.** Replaces the Ionising Radiation (Protection of Persons Undergoing Medical Examination or Treatment) Regulations 1988

**A** **1.**  **A.** true  **B.** false  **C.** false  **D.** true  **E.** true

Increased sensitivity of the rare earth phosphors results in increased speed compared to CaW screens.

Rare earth screens deliver a patient dose 2–3 times lower than CaW screens.

Gadolinium oxysulphide may only be used with orthochromatic film (i.e. one sensitive to green light).

Lanthanum oxybromide emits a line spectrum of blue light, and hence can be used with ordinary X-ray film which is sensitive to ultraviolet (UV) and blue light.

Farr, Allisy-Roberts. *Physics for Medical Imaging*, 1st Edn. W. B. Saunders Co. Ltd.

**A** **2.**  **A.** false  **B.** false  **C.** true  **D.** true  **E.** false

Subject contrast is low.

Skin dose is reduced.

The amount of scattered radiation is relatively high, thus making grids less effective. Hence, the air gap technique is generally preferred.

Efficiency of X-ray production is high, and hence there is decreased heat loading which allows very short exposure times.

Farr, Allisy-Roberts. *Physics for Medical Imaging*, 1st Edn. W. B. Saunders Co. Ltd.

**A** **3.**  **A.** true  **B.** true  **C.** false  **D.** true  **E.** false

The image is minified.

The edges of an image are less bright, less sharp and more distorted, due to difficulty of the electron lens in controlling the peripheral electrons. This is known as vignetting.

Farr, Allisy-Roberts. *Physics for Medical Imaging*, 1st Edn. W. B. Saunders Co. Ltd.

**A 4.** **A.** true **B.** true **C.** false **D.** false **E.** true

Second generation: a narrow fan beam falling on a small curved array of detectors.
Third generation: both the beam and detectors rotate.
Fourth generation: these are of the rotate-still type. The X-ray tube alone rotates with a stationary ring of detectors.
Ring artefacts are most common in third-generation scanners.

Farr, Allisy-Roberts. *Physics for Medical Imaging*, 1st Edn. W. B. Saunders Co. Ltd.

**A 5.** **A.** true **B.** true **C.** false **D.** false **E.** true

The latent image is formed following an exposure and before development.
The speed of an emulsion is largely dependent on the average size of the grains rather than the grain size distribution. The greater the average grain size, the greater the speed of the emulsion.
Film emulsion contains approximately 90% silver bromide and 10% of silver iodide.

Curry, Thomas. *Christensen's Physics of Diagnostic Radiology*, 4th Edn. Williams & Wilkins (Europe) Ltd.

**A 6.** **A.** true **B.** true **C.** true **D.** true **E.** false

The GM counter is able to detect any ionising radiation but does not distinguish between different types, nor can it distinguish between energies of the same radiation.

Curry, Thomas. *Christensen's Physics of Diagnostic Radiology*, 4th Edn. Williams & Wilkins (Europe) Ltd.

**A 7.** **A.** true **B.** true **C.** true **D.** true **E.** false

Whilst both the kVp meter and mA meter are located in the control panel, their connections are in the high-voltage circuit. The high-voltage circuit of an X-ray generator consists of two transformers, an autotransformer and a step-up transformer. The kVp meter is placed in the circuit between the autotransformer and the step-up transformer, and therefore only needs a minimum of insulation when placed in the control panel. However, for the mA meter to provide accurate mA recordings, the connections for the mA meter need to be in the secondary

Exam 10

Answers

coil of the transformer. Hence, the connections need to be grounded.

Armstrong. *Lecture Notes on the Physics of Radiology*, 1st Edn. Clinical Press Ltd., 1990.

**A** 8. **A.** false **B.** false **C.** true **D.** false **E.** true

Attenuation occurs either by absorption of photons, or scattering of photons from the beam.
Attenuation of monochromatic radiation does not change the quality of the radiation. However, the number of the photons in the beam is reduced.
Attenuation of polychromatic radiation is not exponential, i.e. the number of photons remaining in the beam does not decrease by the same percentage with each increment of absorber. When the percentage of transmission is plotted on semi-log paper, it is curved (as opposed to with monochromatic radiation which is a straight line).

Armstrong. *Lecture Notes on the Physics of Radiology*, 1st Edn. Clinical Press Ltd., 1990.

**A** 9. **A.** true **B.** false **C.** true **D.** true **E.** false

The electrostatic image is developed by exposing the surface of the plate to a fine-charged powder called 'toner' which is attracted to the plate surface in proportion to the intensity of the remaining charge. As the toner particles have both positive and negative charges, it is possible to attract either of these selectively to the surface of the plate to produce either a positive or negative image.
The process has very broad exposure latitudes. The resolution is less sensitive to exposure, and hence a single exposure can produce good image resolution in both thick and thin areas of a structure i.e. the breast.

Armstrong. *Lecture Notes on the Physics of Radiology,* 1st Edn. Clinical Press Ltd., 1990.

**A** 10. **A.** false **B.** true **C.** true **D.** true **E.** true

High-ratio grids are more efficient at removing scattered. radiation.

As the bucky factor is the ratio of incident radiation to transmitted radiation, high-ratio grids also have a larger bucky factor. Grid ratio refers to how efficient a grid is at removing secondary (scattered) radiation.

Whilst it is desirable for a grid to only prevent the passage of secondary scattered radiation, there is always some absorption of primary radiation. Hence, when using a grid, exposure factors need to be increased.

Armstrong. *Lecture Notes on the Physics of Radiology*, 1st Edn. Clinical Press Ltd.

**A** **11.** **A.** false **B.** false **C.** true **D.** false **E.** true

The number of electrons in the M shell is 18.
K > L > M. Energy (E):K = 70, E:L = 11, E:M = 2 keV.
Isotopes have identical chemical properties, where A is the mass number and Z is the atomic number.

Farr, Allisy-Roberts. *Physics for Medical Imaging*, 1st Edn. W. B. Saunders Co. Ltd.

**A** **12.** **A.** false **B.** false **C.** false **D.** false **E.** false

With each HVL, the average energy of the photons increases – the beam becomes 'harder' or more penetrating. The second HVL is larger than the first HVL.
The HVL of a typical diagnostic beam is 30 mm.
As an X-ray beam penetrates a material, it becomes progressively more homogenous secondary to beam hardening.
The photoelectric effect results from interactions with 'bound' inner shell electrons.
The probability that the Compton process will occur is proportional to the physical density and in particular electron density, and is inversely proportional to the incident photon energy. It is independent of Z.

Farr, Allisy-Roberts. *Physics for Medical Imaging*, 1st Edn. W. B. Saunders Co. Ltd.

**A** **13.** **A.** true **B.** false **C.** true **D.** false **E.** true

The rating decreases as the kV is increased.
At higher speeds, heat is more evenly spread along the focal track resulting in greater rating.

In continuous fluoroscopy, the rating depends only on the rate of cooling of the tube and not upon focal spot size or type of generator used.
Tube rating is about 35% greater with three-phase generators compared to single-phase generators.

Farr, Allisy-Roberts. *Physics for Medical Imaging*, 1st Edn. W. B. Saunders Co. Ltd.

**A 14. A.** true  **B.** true  **C.** false  **D.** false  **E.** true

A very small focal spot decreases geometric unsharpness.
The air gap technique is usually employed.
There is increased patient dose due to the increased exposure factors required.
Quantum mottle is not increased since the same number of X-ray photons are absorbed in the screen for the same degree of film blackening.

Farr, Allisy-Roberts. *Physics for Medical Imaging*, 1st Edn. W. B. Saunders Co. Ltd.

**A 15. A.** true  **B.** true  **C.** false  **D.** false  **E.** false

Screen efficiency is the proportion of light produced in a screen that reaches the film.
Screen conversion efficiency is 5% for tungstate screens and 20% for rare earth screens.
When using a thicker screen, the same number of X-ray photons are absorbed in the screen for the same film density. Hence, there is no change in noise although resolution is reduced. When the conversion or screen efficiency is increased, a reduced number of X-ray photons are required to be absorbed for the same film density. Hence exposure required and patient dose are reduced, but noise is increased. Increasing screen efficiency reduces resolution but increasing conversion efficiency does not affect resolution. Thus increasing conversion efficiency increases quantum noise but increasing screen thickness does not affect noise; however, both increase the speed of a screen and reduce patient dose.

Farr, Allisy-Roberts. *Physics for Medical Imaging*, 1st Edn. W. B. Saunders Co. Ltd.

**A** **16.** **A.** false   **B.** true   **C.** false   **D.** true   **E.** true

The vidicon tube uses antimony trisulphide as the photoconducting material.
The image intensifier has a 'lag' period of about 1 ms. The camera tube may have a 'lag' of several hundred milliseconds.
50 frames per second is necessary to eliminate flicker altogether.

Farr, Allisy-Roberts. *Physics for Medical Imaging*, 1st Edn. W. B. Saunders Co. Ltd.

**A** **17.** **A.** true   **B.** true   **C.** false   **D.** false   **E.** false

NaI, CsI, CdW may also be used as scintillation crystals in a CT detector.
Scintillation detectors are more sensitive than ionisation chambers.
Ionisation chambers are more stable to voltage fluctuation compared to scintillation detectors.
Ionisation chambers are more suitable for third-generation scanners. Solid state detectors are more appropriate for fourth-generation scanners.

Farr, Allisy-Roberts. *Physics for Medical Imaging*, 1st Edn. W. B. Saunders Co. Ltd.

**A** **18.** **A.** true   **B.** false   **C.** false   **D.** false   **E.** false

Pure metallic silver is deposited on the cathode.
Agitation of either the cathode or the anode brings fresh silver ions closer to the surface of the cathode and increases the yield of pure metallic silver.
It is not possible to recover silver using the electrolytic method; however, silver may be recovered from the wash water using the metallic replacement method.
The electrolytic method requires electrical power, whereas the metallic replacement method involves the use of steel wool only.
Hence, the electrolytic method is considerably more expensive to perform.

Curry, Thomas. *Christensen's Physics of Diagnostic Radiology*, 4th Edn. Williams & Wilkins (Europe) Ltd.

Exam 10

Answers

**A** **19.** **A.** true   **B.** false   **C.** true   **D.** true   **E.** true

Between exposures the voltage falls, and this drop needs to be compensated by recharging the battery from the mains.

Armstrong. *Lecture Notes on the Physics of Radiology*, 1st Edn. Clinical Press Ltd., 1990.

**A** **20.** **A.** true   **B.** false   **C.** true   **D.** false   **E.** false

X-rays, gamma rays, and electrons: 1.
Protons: 5.
Alpha particles: 20.
Neutrons: 5–20 (Energy dependent).

Farr, Allisy-Roberts. *Physics for Medical Imaging*, 1st Edn. W. B. Saunders Co. Ltd.

**A** **21.** **A.** false   **B.** false   **C.** true   **D.** false   **E.** true

Very few operators or practitioners are classified workers.
According to IRR 99, individual dose measurement can be inappropriate for classified workers, and therefore other suitable measurements can be used.
Classified workers, must be aged 18 years or older.

*The Ionising Radiations Regulations 1999.*

**A** **22.** **A.** true   **B.** false   **C.** true   **D.** false   **E.** true

The radiation protection advisor must be consulted, not the RPS, about servicing and correct use of equipment.
Where concentration of activity is low enough the RPA does not need to be consulted.

*The Ionising Radiations Regulations 1999.*

**A** **23.** **A.** true   **B.** false   **C.** false   **D.** false   **E.** true

The annual equivalent dose limit for the skin of a member of the public is 50 mSv.
The five consecutive years dose limit of 100 mSv is only allowed providing the annual effective dose is never greater than 50 mSv.

The annual equivalent dose limit for hands of an employee is 500 mSv.

*The Ionising Radiations Regulations 1999.*

A **24.** **A.** false **B.** true **C.** true **D.** true **E.** false

There is no clear data proving a hereditary genetic effect of radiation exposure.
Stochastic effects may have a long latent period.

Farr, Allisy-Roberts. *Physics for Medical Imaging*, 1st Edn. W. B. Saunders Co. Ltd.

A **25.** **A.** false **B.** true **C.** false **D.** true **E.** true

Schedule 2 of IR(ME)R lists relevant subjects for training.
Patient information detailing the risks associated with ionising radiation must be given to patients undergoing treatment or diagnosis with radioactive medicinal products.

*IR(ME)R 2000.*

**NOTES**

# NOTES

**NOTES**

**NOTES**

# NOTES